Maureen
Marie

Modern Practical Nursing Series

This important nursing series, designed specifically for the State Enrolled Nurse and Pupil Nurse is published as a 'parent' book covering the basic skills entitled AN OUTLINE OF BASIC NURSING CARE, and a number of smaller handbooks covering the individual specialities as the nurse is moved from one discipline to another.

The following volumes are available;
Parent Book: AN OUTLINE OF BASIC NURSING CARE

Elizabeth M Welsh, RGN, RNT.
Director of Nursing and Midwifery Education, Northern Ireland Council for Nurses and Midwives.
Mary Gillespie, RFN, RGN, RCI.
Clinical Instructor, Teaching Division, Glasgow Royal Infirmary and Associated Hospitals.
Catherine Asher, RGN, SCM, RNT.
Senior Nursing Officer, Teaching Division, Glasgow Royal Infirmary and Associated Hospitals.

| 224 pages | 220 illustrations | £1.00 net |

Volume 1: PAEDIATRIC ORTHOPAEDICS

Mary I Gilchrist, RSCN, RGN, ONC.
Ward Sister, Royal Hospital for Sick Children, Drumchapel Branch, Glasgow.
Noel J. Blockey, FRCS, MChOrth.
Consultant Orthopaedic Surgeon, Royal Hospital for Sick Children, Drumchapel Branch, Glasgow.

| 112 pages | 29 illustrations | £0.60 net |

Volume 2: THEATRE ROUTINE

Morag H Campbell, RGN, SCM.
Senior Nursing Officer (Theatres & CSSD), Glasgow Royal Infirmary.

| 160 pages | 69 illustrations | £0.60 net |

Volume 3: PAEDIATRIC SURGERY

Elizabeth D Strathdee, SRN, RSCN.
Ward Sister, Royal Hospital for Sick Children, Glasgow.
D G Young, MB, ChB, FRCS. (Edin), DTM & H.
Senior Lecturer in Paediatric Surgery, The University, Glasgow.
Honorary Consultant Surgeon, Royal Hospital for Sick Children, Glasgow.

| 96 pages | 30 illustrations | £0.60 net |

Volume 4: DERMATOLOGY

A Keenan, RGN, SCM.
Ward Sister, Glasgow Royal Infirmary.
J O'D Alexander, MB, ChB, FRCP.
Consultant Dermatologist, Glasgow Royal Infirmary.

| 96 pages | 34 black & white, 24 colour illustrations | £0.75 net |

Volume 5: UROLOGY

Margaret W A Stirling, RGN, SCM.
Ward Sister, Urological Department, Glasgow Royal Infirmary.
Roy Scott, MB, ChB, FRCS. (Glas.), FRCS, (Ed).
Consultant Urologist, Glasgow Royal Infirmary.

| 80 pages | 17 illustrations | £0.65 net |

Volume 6: PLASTIC SURGERY AND BURNS TREATMENT

Ian T Jackson, MB, ChB, FRCS. (Glas.), FRCS. (Ed).
Consultant Plastic Surgeon, Glasgow & West of Scotland Regional Plastic and Oral
Surgery Service, Canniesburn Hospital, Bearsden, Glasgow.
E S Macallan, RGN, SCM, Plastic Surgery Cert.
Former Ward Sister, Glasgow and West of Scotland Regional Plastic and Oral Surgery
Service, Canniesburn Hospital, Bearsden, Glasgow. At present a member of the Teaching
Staff in the School of Nursing, Glasgow Royal Infirmary and Associated Hospitals.

160 pages   90 illustrations   £0.60 net

Volume 7: PSYCHIATRY

Emily A Lee, RGN, RMN, RCI. (Edin).
Glasgow Royal Infirmary and Associated Hospitals Teaching Department, Clinical
Instructor based at Eastern District Hospital, Glasgow.
A B Sclare, MB, ChB, FRCP. (Glas), FRCP. (Edin), MRCP. (Lond), DPM.
Consultant Psychiatrist, Eastern District Hospital and Glasgow Royal Infirmary,
Mackintosh Lecturer in Psychological Medicine, University of Glasgow.

192 pages   £0.60 net

Volume 8: ORTHOPAEDIC SURGERY

Thomas H Norton, MB, ChB, FRCSE.
Consultant Orthopaedic Surgeon to Victoria Infirmary and Philipshill Orthopaedic
Hospital, Glasgow.
Judith M Tait, SCM, ONC, RNT.
Senior Nursing Officer, Teaching Division, Glasgow Royal Infirmary School of Nursing.

148 pages   128 two-colour illustrations   £0.90 net

Volume 9: ADULT MEDICINE

E H R Laird, RGN, SCM, HV Cert.
Unit Nursing Officer, Glasgow Royal Infirmary.
R D Barr, MB, ChB, MRCP.
Registrar, Medical Department, Glasgow Royal Infirmary.

144 pages   21 illustrations   £0.65 net

Volume 10: ADULT SURGERY

A McWee, RGN, SCM.
Glasgow Royal Infirmary School of Nursing.
M Kennedy Browne, BSc, MD, FRCSE.
Consultant Surgeon, Glasgow Royal Infirmary.

224 pages   128 illustrations   £1.00 net

Volume 11: MEDICAL PAEDIATRICS

William B Doig, MB, ChB, MRCP, DCH.
Consultant Paediatric Cardiologist, Royal Hospital for Sick Children, Glasgow.
Alison Montford, RSCN, RGN.
Formerly Ward Sister, Royal Hospital for Sick Children, Glasgow.

168 pages   74 illustrations   £0.95 net

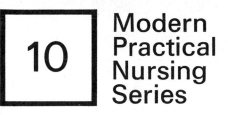

10 Modern Practical Nursing Series

Adult Surgery

A.C. McWee, R.G.N., S.C.M., R.N.T.
*Senior Nursing Officer, Teaching Division,
Glasgow Royal Infirmary and Associated Hospitals.*

M. Kennedy Browne, B.Sc., M.D., F.R.C.S.E.
Consultant Surgeon, Glasgow Royal Infirmary.

WILLIAM HEINEMAN MEDICAL BOOKS LIMITED
23 Bedford Square London WC1B 3HT

First Published 1972
©A.C. McWee and M. Kennedy Browne
Illustrations by Jean Macdonald and Frank B. Price
ISBN 0 433 20700 0

Printed in Great Britain by
Redwood Press Limited, Trowbridge, Wiltshire .

CONTENTS

INTRODUCTION

Surgery is an ancient craft. Records of many primitive civilisations include reference to simple surgical operations mainly relating to the letting out of demons or spirits, while in more advanced civilisations cutting "for the stone", relieving an abscess, or the letting of blood was common. Indeed the surgeon belonged to the arts and crafts rather than to the sciences until the eighteenth century, at which time in England, surgery was the prerogative of the barbers, hence their red and white pole representing blood and bandages. In that era, however surgery parted from the realm of the barbers and became allied to the rest of medicine and became a science as well as an art and craft. Today the surgeon deals with many conditions by the same techniques and drugs as the physician. He is nevertheless characterised by the fact that he operates and cuts into the patient in order to alleviate his suffering. The conditions with which the surgeon is concerned fall broadly under three headings. First of all are the mechanical conditions. These may take the form of congenital malformations, or they may be acquired mechanical conditions such as blockages of the bowel, twisting of the bowel, or swallowed foreign bodies. Also under this heading comes the treatment of trauma in its widest sense, it may be the orthopaedic surgeon repairing broken bones, the neuro-surgeon dealing with head injuries or a general surgeon repairing ruptured organs and vessels. Training for this calls for all the surgical skills.

The second indication for surgery is inflammatory conditions. These may be infections characterised by suppuration where the time honoured method of letting "out the pus" is all too often required while some inflamed organs by their position or by their nature require removal rather than treatment by drugs.

Lastly, the tumours, which call for the most radical surgery if the disease is to be eliminated.

Unlike other branches of medicine, in surgery events move quickly — the patient often requires operation without undue loss of time and thereafter usually recovers very quickly. Complications, if they do

1

arise, also occur quickly, and the most common of these is haemorrhage. This often requires immediate treatment. Indeed, this is an instance where the nurse's role is paramount since the surgeon is unlikely to be there in person when the complication occurs. The nurse must know the signs of impending danger and not only alert the medical staff but be able to take the first steps in dealing with the situation. Because of the nature of surgery the nursing and medical staff must work in the closest co-operation as a team. It is most demanding both physically and mentally but at the same time most rewarding.

The following book gives an outline of the nursing care carried out in surgical wards and a synopsis of some of the commoner surgical conditions. The latter are included since it is felt that it is easier to understand surgical nursing if one knows what has been done in theatre and why it has been done.

1
An Outline of the Structure and Function of the Human Body

The study of the way in which the body is built (anatomy) and the way in which it works (physiology) is not only of interest to a nurse, but it is essential that she understands the normal workings before she can understand what happens to the body should it be diseased. It is the purpose of this short section to outline the anatomy and physiology of the body as a whole and stress a little the particular sections to which reference will be made in later chapters when diseases of the various organs are discussed.

The Cells and Tissues

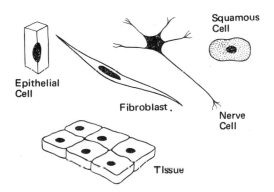

Squamous Cell

Epithelial Cell

Fibroblast .

Nerve Cell

Tissue

The human body is made up of millions of cells of different kinds, shapes and sizes. A cell is the basic unit from which the body is built but is so small that you would require a microscope to see it. Cells of the same type are stuck together or arranged together to form tissues. Cells and tissues making up the body are living structures and therefore require oxygen and nourishment so that they may live and they must have the ability to get rid of the waste substances which are produced when the nourishment and the oxygen are used by the cells. The tissues are of four main types:—

1. Epithelial tissue
2. Connective tissue
3. Muscle tissue
4. Nervous tissue

1. Epithelial Tissue

Epithelial tissue is found covering the outside of the body in the form of the skin and inside the body it lines and covers the tubes and the organs, for example, inside the blood vessel a very smooth, delicate lining is required and in the lungs a very thin wall to allow oxygen to pass through is needed. In various parts of the body cells are arranged to form membranes. The digestive tract is lined by a mucous membrane which produces a slimy substance called mucus. Lining some of the joints, another membrane, called synovial membrane is found, which produces a very sticky substance called synovial fluid. The large body cavities are lined by a serous membrane which produces a watery fluid called serous fluid. The serous membrane in the thorax is called the pleura, in the abdominal cavity, the peritoneum.

2. Connective Tissue

Connective tissue connects or supports other tissues and organs of the body. This type of tissue includes such things as fat, bone, cartilage, fibrous tissue, elastic tissue and areolar or packing tissue.

3. Muscle Tissue

Muscle tissue is the tissue which allows organs and the body to move. It has the ability to contract and relax. When it is attached to the skeleton it is called skeletal muscle or voluntary muscle. When it is making up the wall of an organ inside the body it is called involuntary muscle and the muscle which makes up the wall of the heart is called cardiac muscle.

4

4. Nervous Tissue

Nervous tissue is very highly specialised tissue and it carries instructions and information to and from the various organs and parts of the body.

These tissues are arranged in layers or patterns to form the organs of the body and the structures which support them.

Systems

When several organs work in conjunction with one another, this is called a system. There are nine systems in the body.

1. Skeletal
2. Muscular
3. Respiratory
4. Circulatory
5. Digestive
6. Excretory
7. Endocrine
8. Nervous
9. Reproductive

Cavities

The organs and structures forming the various systems are found in the cavities of the body.

The Cranial Cavity
The *cranial cavity* is the space in which the brain is housed in the head.

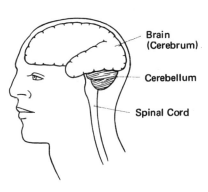

Brain (Cerebrum)

Cerebellum

Spinal Cord

The Thoracic Cavity

The *thoracic cavity* or thorax, is in the upper part of the trunk and contains the air passages, the lungs, the heart and some of the large blood vessels. The floor of the thoracic cavity is made of the diaphragm, the walls consist of the ribs and the muscles lying between the ribs.

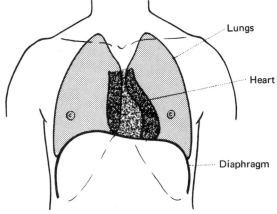

Lungs

Heart

Diaphragm

The Abdominal Cavity

The *abdominal cavity* lies in the lower part of the trunk directly under the diaphragm, which forms its roof.

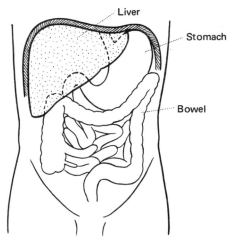

Liver

Stomach

Bowel

The walls of the abdominal cavity are made mainly of muscle. The organs found in the abdominal cavity are the kidneys, the stomach, and intestine, the spleen, the liver, the gall bladder and the adrenal glands.

The Pelvic Cavity

The *pelvic cavity* is the lowest part or the lowest cavity situated in the trunk. Its walls are made of the bones of the pelvis and the organs contained in it are the bladder, the reproductive organs and the lower part of the intestine.

The limbs, that is the arms and legs, consist of bones, muscles, nerves, blood vessels and of course are covered in skin. The head is connected to the trunk by the neck and in it are air and food passages and part of the spinal column.

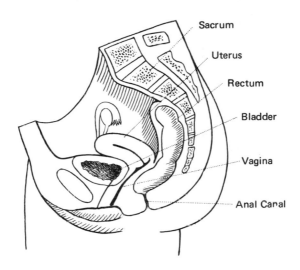

Sacrum

Uterus

Rectum

Bladder

Vagina

Anal Canal

Other Areas and Hollows

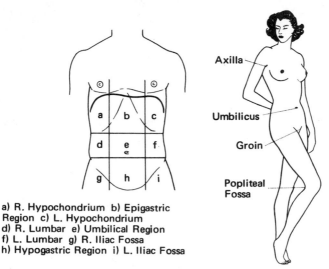

a) R. Hypochondrium b) Epigastric Region c) L. Hypochondrium
d) R. Lumbar e) Umbilical Region
f) L. Lumbar g) R. Iliac Fossa
h) Hypogastric Region i) L. Iliac Fossa

Axilla

Umbilicus

Groin

Popliteal Fossa

Special names are given to some areas and hollows in the body. The armpit is called the axilla (plural, axillae); the hollows between the trunk and legs, the groins; the hollows behind the knees, the popliteal spaces; the umbilicus is the name given to the scar or navel near the centre of the abdomen where the baby's cord was attached before birth. The areas of the abdomen are named as shown on the accompanying diagram.

Skeletal and Muscular Systems

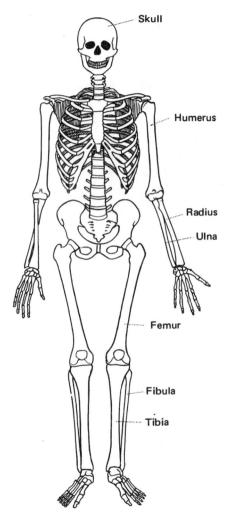

The bones form the skeleton which makes the framework for the body.

Muscular Systems

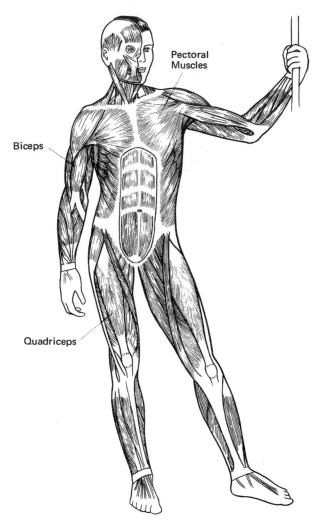

Pectoral
Muscles

Biceps

Quadriceps

Attached to it are the skeletal muscles or muscular system which is
responsible for moving the body.

Some Important Muscles

Anterior Abdominal Wall

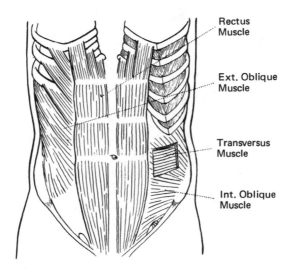

Rectus Muscle

Ext. Oblique Muscle

Transversus Muscle

Int. Oblique Muscle

The anterior abdominal wall is important because it is through this wall that many operations are performed. The wall is made up of 4 layers of muscle tissue arranged in different directions and covered by skin. It is a very strong wall of muscle and supports the abdominal organs, allows some of the spine movements, assists in breathing, coughing and sneezing, and is involved in the emptying of the bladder (micturition), and the emptying of the bowel (defaecation). Although, generally speaking, the anterior abdominal wall is very strong, there are three places in it where, because of the structure, it is slightly weaker. These are the inguinal canals, the femoral canals and the umbilicus. The inguinal canals are small tunnels in the muscle wall, found one on either side, just about the level of the hip bone, and the femoral canals are little openings found in the muscle of each groin below the level of the inguinal canals.

Diaphragm

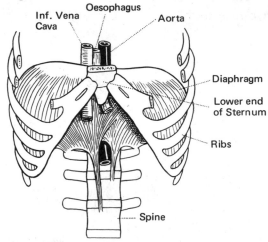

The diaphragm is the sheet of muscle which separates the thoracic cavity from the abdominal cavity. It is shaped rather like a dome or the lid of an old fashioned bread bin. There are openings in the diaphragm through which the biggest artery in the body, called the aorta, passes and the biggest vein, called the inferior vena cava, also passes and the tube which carries the food from the mouth to the stomach, called the oesophagus. When the diaphragm contracts it flattens and air is pulled into the lungs through the air passages and when the diaphragm relaxes it returns to its normal dome shape and the air rushes out from the lungs.

Intercostal Muscles

The intercostal muscles lie between the ribs. When the intercostal muscles contract the overall size of the thoracic cavity is increased therefore more air enters the lungs. Both the diaphragm and the intercostal muscles are therefore important because they are the main muscles of breathing. The name given to breathing is respiration.

Breathing in is called inspiration. Breathing out is called expiration.

Respiration is the process by which air is moved in and out of the lungs.

The Respiratory System

Oxygen is vital to the life of each individual cell in the body and therefore it is vital to the human being. Oxygen is found in the atmosphere and the organs making up the respiratory system are responsible for enabling this oxygen to get into the blood and waste gases to be released from the blood into the atmosphere. The passage-way from the nose into the lungs must be kept clear otherwise death will result. Air is breathed into the nose and from there passes into the pharynx which is shared by the digestive tract. At the lower end of the pharynx the tube continues as the larynx and from this, as the trachea. The trachea divides two tubes called bronchi one of which goes to each lung. All these tubes are collectively referred to as the air passages. While the air passes through these air passages it is filtered so that any dust in it is removed, it is moistened and it is warmed by the many blood vessels found in the walls of these tubes. The tonsils which are made of protective tissue called lymphoid tissue are found in the pharynx. The vocal cords which allow us to speak are in the larynx. The lungs are made of branches of the bronchi forming smaller air passages within the lungs and as these tubes become smaller they end in little dilated thin walled sacs called alveoli. All the alveoli and small air passages are closely surrounded by blood vessels and supported by connective tissue. The lungs are covered by a serous membrane called the pleura. The exchange of gases from the blood and air takes place in the alveoli. To draw air into the lungs the intercostal muscles and the diaphragm must contract and air is pulled in and when these muscles relax the air rushes out of the lungs. This mechanism is controlled automatically by nerves but is under the control of the will, during speaking or singing.

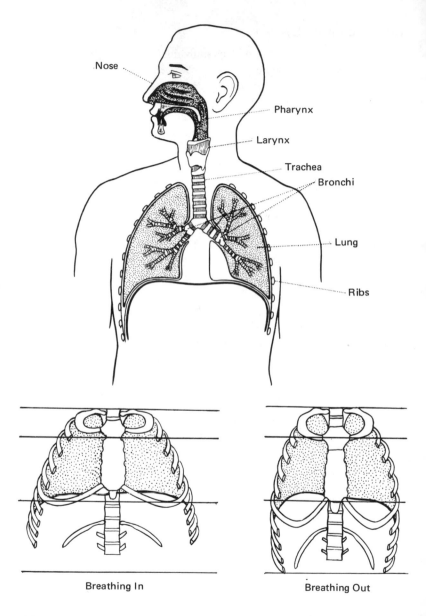

Nose

Pharynx

Larynx

Trachea

Bronchi

Lung

Ribs

Breathing In

Breathing Out

The Circulatory System

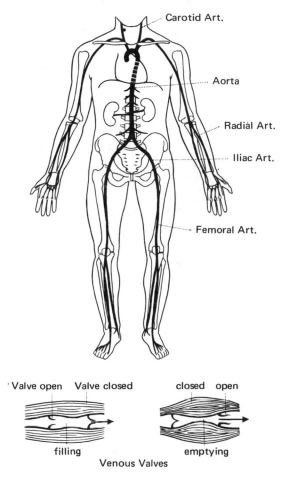

Carotid Art.

Aorta

Radial Art.

Iliac Art.

Femoral Art.

Valve open   Valve closed   closed   open

filling   emptying

Venous Valves

The circulatory system consists of a double sided muscular pump called the heart and a series of tubes which carry the blood. The tubes carrying the blood from the heart are called arteries and carrying the blood to the heart are called veins. There are very small tubes with very thin walls called capillaries which join the arteries to the veins.

It is through the thin wall of the capillaries that nourishment escapes to supply the cells, and waste gains entrance to the blood for ultimate excretion. The wall of the artery is mainly muscle and connective tissue and is lined with a very smooth, delicate lining. The veins also have have connective and muscle tissue in their structure with a smooth lining but their wall is relatively thinner. Many of the veins also have valves as these are required to assist the blood back to the heart, for example, from the feet and legs where the blood is returning against the force of gravity. The squeezing action of the muscles when they contract and relax also helps the blood to return to the heart.

Blood is the fluid which flows in the circulatory system. It contains plasma which is the fluid part of the blood and the cells which float in the plasma. The plasma has various substances dissolved in it including the nutrient materials, amino acids, glucose, vitamins, fatty acids. It also contains salts, waste substances from tissue work, hormones, protective substances and dissolved gases such as oxygen, carbon dioxide and nitrogen. The plasma also contains substances which will be activated and cause clotting if there is any damage to the blood vessel. There are three types of cells in the blood —

1. Red blood cells
2. White blood cells
3. Platelets

The red blood cells are important because they carry the oxygen in the substance called haemoglobin.

The white blood cells are of various types but are important in the protection of the body because they have the ability to destroy micro-organisms.

The platelets are very small cells necessary in the process of clotting.

The functions of the blood therefore are —

1. To carry oxygen and nourishment to the cells
2. To carry carbon dioxide from the cells to the respiratory system for excretion
3. To carry waste products away from the cells.

It also has the ability to clot and thus help to control haemorrhage if the blood vessel is damaged in any way, and is able to fight infection.

The Digestive System

The gastro intestinal tract and associated organs are collectively called the digestive system. This system is responsible for receiving food and breaking it down.

1. Using chemical substances (enzymes) from the glands around the tract

2. By the movement of the various parts of the intestinal tract.

The tract extends from the mouth to the anus and is a tube which varies in shape and size depending on what function the particular part has to fulfil. The tract has a very good blood supply, since food, once it is broken down, has to be absorbed into the blood stream.

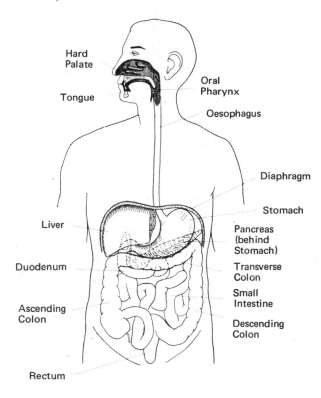

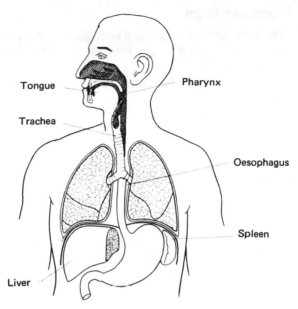

Tongue

Pharynx

Trachea

Oesophagus

Spleen

Liver

Mouth and Oesophagus

At the upper end of the tract is the mouth which is the cavity where food is received. As it is bitten and chewed by the teeth it is mixed with a watery secretion called saliva which comes from the salivary glands situated around the mouth. The saliva keeps the mouth clean and moist, moistens food, and lubricates it making swallowing easier.

The tongue is a very agile muscle covered by a special roughened surface containing taste buds. The tongue helps to mix the food and assists in swallowing.

Behind the nose and mouth is a tube called the pharynx. Leading from the pharynx is a tube going to the lungs and also a muscular tube called the oesophagus which passes down through the thoracic cavity to the stomach. In the oesophagus food is moved down by movement called peristalsis. Peristalsis is a movement in which muscle contracts behind the food and relaxes in front of it and so pushes into a dilated muscular bag called the stomach.

Stomach and Small Intestine

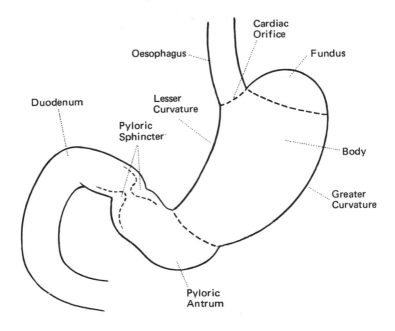

The stomach lies below the diaphragm in the upper left hand side of the abdominal cavity and it acts mainly as a food reservoir. The opening into the stomach is called the cardiac orifice and the opening from the stomach into the small intestine is called the pylorus and is closed by a muscle called the pyloric sphincter. The lining of the stomach is made of mucous membrane which produces mucus. Glands in the stomach produce gastric juice which is acid and contains enzymes which, with muscle movements of the stomach, help to break down the food to a simpler form. The acid also helps to kill micro-organisms. The stomach produces a substance which is needed before vitamin B.12 can be absorbed. This vitamin is eventually used in the bone marrow to produce red blood cells.

The small intestine is a muscular tube coiled up in the abdominal cavity. It is the part of the gastro intestinal tract which continues after the stomach and is divided into three parts

1. the duodenum
2. the jejunum
3. the ileum.

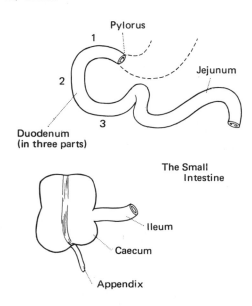

The Small Intestine

The duodenum curves round the head of the pancreas from which a juice called pancreatic juice is poured into the duodenum to help in the digestion of food. Bile produced in the liver, stored in the gall bladder and passed down the common bile duct enters the duodenum and also assists in digestion. In the lining of the small intestine there are glands producing intestinal juice. The peristaltic movement of the intestine and the action of enzymes further breaks down the food and after all this treatment it is mostly ready for absorption through the walls of the ileum into the blood stream. The ileum leads into the large intestine and the opening between the small and the large intestine is controlled by a valve called the ileocaecal valve.

The Large Intestine

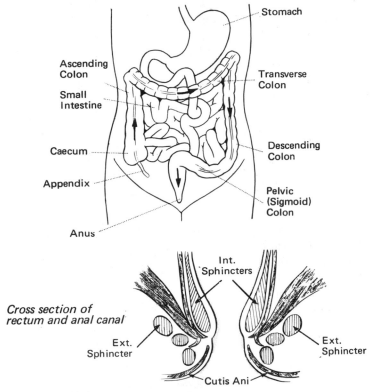

The large intestine, a muscular tube with a wider lumen than the small intestine, is also called the colon. The muscle is in two layers, one running round the intestine, the other along it. There are several different parts of the large intestine. These are the caecum to the lower end of which is attached the appendix, the sigmoid colon, the ascending colon, the transverse colon, the descending colon, the rectum and the anal canal. The anal canal has a ring shaped muscle at the end of it called internal and external sphincters. The position of each of these parts may be seen in the accompanying diagram. In the lining of the large intestine there are small glands which produce mucus. The function of the large intestine is to allow the absorption of water from the intestinal contents into the blood stream. There are micro-organisms normally present in the large intestine which help to break down indigestible foodstuffs. Movement of a slower kind takes place in the large intestine and moves the contents along as far as the rectum. When the rectum is full, nerves are stimulated and the person is made aware of this fact. The rectum contracts, the internal sphincter relaxes and the external spincter is relaxed at will and the abdominal muscles contract and assist in the expulsion of the waste material (faeces), to the exterior. The whole process of expulsion of faeces is called defaecation.

The parts of the digestive system found in the abdominal cavity are either supported or slung in a fold of peritoneum. The name, mesentry, is given to the fold of peritoneum which slings most of the small intestine from the posterior abdominal wall.

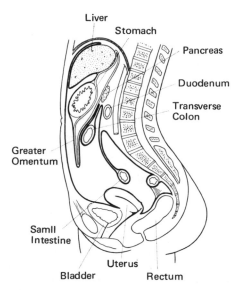

Once the foods have been reduced to a form suitable for absorption into the blood stream they are as follows —

        Carbohydrate has been converted to glucose
        protein to amino acids
        fat is in the form of fatty acids.

Once absorbed these food stuffs plus the salts and the water are carried in veins from the gastro intestinal tract to the liver.

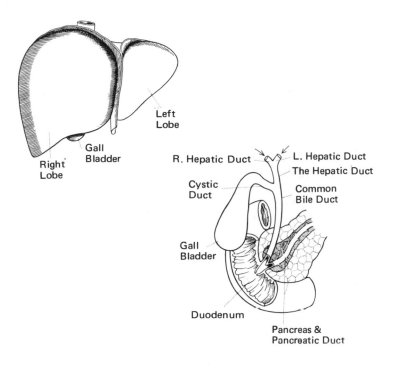

The system of veins through which they pass is called the
portal system. It delivers this very rich blood to the liver which
is a large gland in the upper right hand corner of the abdominal
cavity. The liver is a very active gland. It makes bile from broken
down red blood cells. The bile is then stored in a little pear shaped
muscular bag on the under side of the liver called the gall bladder.
After it has been stored and concentrated, the bile travels from
the gall bladder down through a duct called the common bile duct,
into the duodenum where it helps to digest fats. The liver also stores
some of the vitamins, iron, and glucose; and prepares the amino
acids and fat for use by the cells of the body. Because the liver is
such an active structure it produces a large amount of heat.

The Systems which Excrete Waste

Respiratory System

As mentioned above the respiratory system excretes waste gases.

Urinary System

The urinary system, consisting of the kidneys, the ureters, the bladder and the urethra are responsible for removing excess fluid and waste substances from the blood and passing them first of all into the bladder for storage and from there the waste is expelled from the body via the urethra. There is a sphincter at the base of the bladder which is not under the control of the will and this is called the internal sphincter. The external sphincter at a lower level in the urethra is under the control of the will. When the bladder is full the nervous system makes the individual aware of this situation and an impulse to empty the bladder is felt. The internal sphincter automatically relaxes and if the time is convenient the external sphincter is relaxed at will and urine, which is the waste from the kidneys, is voided. The expulsion of this waste from the body is assisted by the contraction not only of the bladder but also of the anterior abdominal wall and diaphragm and the process of emptying is called micturition.

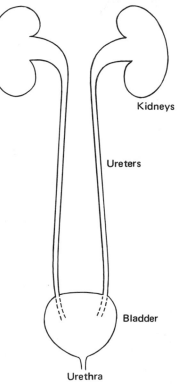

Kidneys

Ureters

Bladder

Urethra

Skin

A limited amount of waste and water is excreted in sweat from the skin.

2
The Controlling Systems

Nervous Systems

The nervous system which consists of the brain, the spinal cord and the nerves which travel to and from all the organs and structures making up the human body, helps to control the way in which the body functions.

Information received by the brain travels along nerves which are called sensory nerves. These travel from —

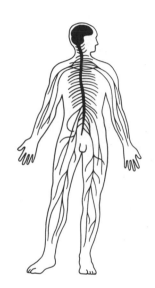

1. The skin which sends information regarding pain, pressure temperature and touch.

2. The eyes, the ears, the nose and the tongue send stimuli which the brain interprets as sight, sound, smell and taste.

3. The joints and the muscles also send information about their position.

4. The ear sends information about the position of the head in space.

Instructions from the brain travel along nerves which are called motor nerves and these stimulate some action in a structure or organ of the body.

Endocrine System

The endocrine or glandular system also assists in control. It is formed by glands in various parts of the body which produce chemical substances called hormones which travel in the blood and cause activity in other organs.

The pituitary gland which lies at the base of the brain secretes several hormones which affect the functioning of the other endocrine glands and also the growth of the body.

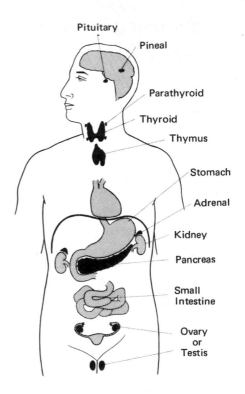

The thyroid gland is situated in the neck and the hormone from this controls the rate at which the whole body functions. Situated behind the thyroid gland are the parathyroid glands which secrete a hormone which governs the use of calcium in the body.

Sitting on the top of each kidney is an adrenal gland. The inner part of this gland produces adrenaline which helps us to cope with stressful situations and the outer part produces hormones called steroids and one of the important steroid hormones is called cortisone.

The pancreas is found in the abdominal cavity slightly behind the stomach and in the curve of the duodenum. It produces a hormone called insulin which controls the use of carbohydrate in the body.

The Female Reproductive System

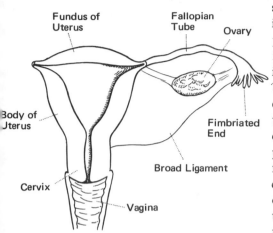

Fundus of Uterus

Fallopian Tube

Ovary

Body of Uterus

Fimbriated End

Broad Ligament

Cervix

Vagina

The reproductive system in the female is partly external and partly internal. Inside is the womb or uterus in which the child grows before it is born. On either side of this are the female sex glands called ovaries which product the ovum (the female sex cell). The cell is then carried in one of the two uterine tubes from the ovary to the uterus.

Under the influence of hormones excreted by the ovary, the lining of the uterus thickens each month in preparation for pregnancy. If pregnancy does not occur the lining is cast off in what is called menstruation. The cycle of building up this lining and its eventual shedding is called the menstrual cycle and the series of events which take place in the uterus generally occur about every 28 days from teenage to middle-age. The external organs are collectively called the vulva and consist of two large folds and two smaller folds of tissue called labia. These are lined with mucous membrane. The tube which connects the external organs to the internal organs is called the vagina. This is the tube along which the child passes when it is being born.

The Breast

The breast is an accessory organ to the female reproductive system. There are two breasts which are situated on the anterior chest wall.

They consist of glandular and connective tissue which is active only during pregnancy and when a baby is being fed. The breasts are small in a child, develop as a person matures and shrink in old age. The structure also includes fat which lies mainly under the skin of the breast and it is this that determines their size. The ducts from the glandular tissue lead to, and open on to, the surface of the breast at a small elevation in the centre called the nipple. Hormones from the pituitary gland control the secretion of milk from the breast.

Male Reproductive System

Most of the male reproductive system is contained in a pouch which is suspended from the perineum which is the area between the legs and this pouch is called the scrotum. Inside this pouch are the male sex glands called the testes and during the mature years the testes produce the male sex cells called spermatazoa and the male sex hormone. The spermatazoa are transported via a complicated system of tubes to the urethra which passes through the perineum and penis. The male urethra provides a passage for the secretion from lubricating glands and spermatozoa as well as for urine.

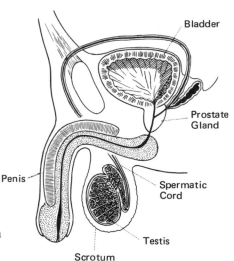

THE SURGICAL SITUATION

Team work is the essence of patient care. To be successful in sport each member of a team must play his part. Although the importance of each member may vary from time to time, the ultimate success in any game is achieved only if each team member fulfils his function and co-operates with his team mates.

The surgical team consists, not only of the people who come into direct contact with the patient, such as doctors and nurses, but also, of those who work in specialised departments and laboratories such as Radiologists, Bacteriologists and Pathologists, whose work indirectly influences the patients' care.

The nurse, as part of this team, has a big responsibility for the safety and care of the patient while in Hospital. It is her duty to make sure that the patient is given a high standard of nursing care and that during his stay in the ward, is not harmed in any way. There are two problems giving rise to particular concern in a surgical ward; the first is that of patient identification, and secondly that of infection.

Identification

The patient may at some time during his stay be unconscious due to illness or anaesthesia, or be drowsy as a result of medication prior to operation. In all these situations he is at risk, as he is unable to identify himself adequately and since the turnover of patients in the surgical wards has increased greatly in recent years the problem of identification is one of the utmost importance.

To overcome this problem the patient may have a plastic identification bracelet attached to his wrist. These bracelets are of various types, and have been produced with the following characteristics.

1. They are not easily removed, a feature necessary for the restless, disorientated patient or a curious child.

2. They contain readable particulars of name, ward and hospital number, which must correspond with all other records, such as chart or case sheet.

3. They are waterproof to ensure that the information remains readable.

4. They conform comfortably to different wrist sizes.

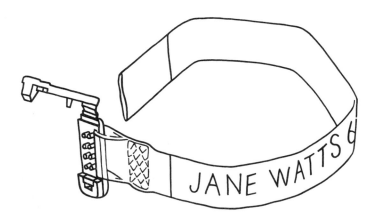

The nurse should always check the patient's identity prior to any treatments or administration of drugs or blood and the bracelet is very useful if the patient is unable to communicate in the ordinary way. The bracelet is also valuable in the operation situation as it can be used as a means of identification of the individual and thus prevent a possible wrong operation being performed.

Infection

The second problem is that of infection, which will be considered in a general sense and then with particular reference to the hospital situation.

Micro-organisms

A micro-organism is a living structure which, on entering the body, may cause disease. When a micro-organism capable of causing disease enters the body and multiplies in it, or part of it, the body is said to be infected. Micro-organisms are so small that it is necessary to use a microscope to see them. They are therefore particularly dangerous as infection can take place without the nurse being aware of it. In the hospital when a patient's resistance is perhaps lowered, the patient is more liable to infection. Normally a healthy, unbroken skin helps to repel micro-organisms, but if there is a break, as with a surgical incision, micro-organisms have a better opportunity to enter the body.

When a man goes on a journey he can leave the country from various points and take a land, sea or air route to reach his destination. On arrival he can enter the country of his choice at several different points and may settle in one town or move around. The journey of the micro-organism from its normal habitat is rather like this. Its normal abode is called the source. This may be within the patient's own body, for example, some micro-organisms are normally present in the bowel, but if these move into the urinary tract they cause infection. Alternatively the source may be in another person, animal or in the soil.

Micro-organisms leave a person or animal in discharges such as urine, faeces, pus, sputum, nasal or oral secretions. Just as man can travel in various ways so can the micro-organisms. They may travel in droplets, from coughing or speaking, which are sprayed into the air or land in the dust. Sometimes the discharges contaminate things like toys, bed linen, and china. If these are in touch with another person he may become infected. Through faulty hygiene the micro-organisms may also contaminate food or drink and again can cause infection.

Man can enter a country at various points, similarly micro-organisms can gain entry to the body in various ways. They may be breathed in from dust stirred up at bedmaking or sweeping, be inhaled from droplets suspended in the air, be swallowed in food or drink, enter through a cut or break in the skin or be introduced into the body on contaminated instruments, needles or catheters. A few infections can be introduced if an infected insect (for example a mosquito) bites a person. Some micro-organisms are spread by direct contact and a good example of this is venereal disease. Once the infection has entered the body it may stay in one place (e.g. in a wound) or spread to other parts of the body (e.g. septicaemia).

A country is protected at all times from undesirable entrants or goods by customs and immigration officials. Similarly in the body

1. The intact skin acts as a mechanical barrier

2. The stomach secretions are harmful to some micro-organisms and the sticky mucus produced in various parts of the body hinders the entrance of micro-organisms.

3. Within the blood the white blood cells help to protect the body by dealing with any micro-organisms which might invade.

If a country is invaded more troops are mobilised, likewise in the body, if virulent micro-organisams attack, the body's reaction to the infection is much greater, therefore, there is an increased blood supply to the particular part and the part becomes hot, red and swollen.

Infection can be stopped from spreading by attacking it at the source of infection, or on its route to or at the patient himself. The source can perhaps be removed, isolated or destroyed. En route, measures such as handwashing and the use of sterile articles may stop the spread. The infected patient may be treated with antibiotics.

Cross Infection

A particular kind of infection which is important in hospital is cross infection. This means that a person admitted with one illness becomes infected by micro-organisms from some other source while in hospital. The source may be a doctor, nurse, domestic or other member of staff working in the ward, visitor or another patient.

There are several measures which can be taken to overcome cross infection. The personal hygience of each individual having any contact with the patient, must be of the highest standard. This can only be achieved if staff

1. Have sufficient numbers of uniform to allow for adequate laundering

2. Have adequate changing accommodation with sufficient toilet and washing facilities

3. Realise the importance of a high standard of personal hygiene.

Infection from the skin (particularly of the hands), from wounds and from the upper respiratory tract, can be spread from staff or patient to another patient. No member of staff who has an infection, whether it be influenza or skin sepsis, should be working in a surgical ward. All small cuts or abrasions should be covered. Hands should be washed, not scrubbed, as the latter can damage the nurse's skin.

They should always be dried thoroughly, preferably using disposable towels, as moisture can damage skin and is a facility enjoyed by the micro-organism. The hair of members of staff, whether male or female, must be kept clean and neatly groomed at all times as it can harbour micro-organisms. If not, while the nurse works with patients infection can be spread. Staff should at all times be encouraged to use paper handkerchiefs. There should be adequate means for disposal of these.

The patient's hygiene may or may not be attended to by the Nurse, but she is responsible for making sure that it is adequate at all times. Bedpans, urinals, and sanitary annexes must be kept scrupulously clean. Soiled linen must be handled as little as possible as it may be contaminated by micro-organisms from a wound or from the bowel. The use of disposable equipment, e.g. spatulae and sputum cartons, helps to overcome cross infection providing there are adequate disposal facilities.

Although in many wards nowadays, it is the responsibility of a domestic supervisor to make sure that cleaning of the ward is carried out, nurses have a responsibility to indicate to the supervisor if the standard of work, in her eyes, is not high enough and will have an adverse effect on the patients. A ward which is purpose built and properly designed should have no unnecessary ledges, crannies, and corners in which dust can collect. Any cleaning of floors should be done with a vacuum and any dusting should be damp dusting. To make sure that there is no unnecessary dust rising from the bed, pillows and mattresses should be adequately covered (perhaps with a fine plastic cover). Bed linen should be handled carefully at all times and should not be flapped around unnecessarily as this causes dust to fly. Bed linen must never be passed or put from one bed to another, as this is one sure way of spreading infection. Beds should be adequately spaced with about eight feet from bed centre to bed centre to ensure that infection does not spread easily. A surgical ward should be well ventilated without draughts.

Flies and insects should be excluded from a surgical ward. Modern aerosols, properly used, can deal with this.

The kitchen of a surgical ward, like any kitchen, should always be kept spotlessly clean. Food being stored in the refrigerator should be kept in covered containers. The food refrigerator should be used only for storing food and not for example to store blood, as this is dangerous. Urine specimens, wound swabs and specimens of sputum must never, under any conditions be put into the ward food 'fridge'.

So far, the measures suggested have been general ones. Special measures would be used in particular situations.

1. During dressings
2. While assisting doctor at procedures using an aseptic technique.

The term "asepsis" is used to denote the absence of micro-organisms and a technique on this principle requires that all instruments and dressings which are used must be sterile. If an article is sterile it is free from living micro-organisms and spores.

Sterilisation

Most micro-organisms require warmth, moisture and a supply of food to grow and multiply. If these conditions are not available some micro-organisms die but others go into a "resting phase" till conditions are again suitable. When in this state they develop a protective covering and are called spores. These are very difficult to kill so that any method of sterilisation must be capable of destroying ordinary micro-organisms and the spores. The commoner methods used in hospital are boiling, autoclaving, dry heat, gamma radiation and the use of chemicals.

Boiling

Boiling is an inefficient method of sterilising as the five minutes which kills many micro-organisms does not kill spores. It involves the use of Cheatles or Basin forceps for removing the items from boiling water. These must be kept in a container of antiseptic solution. The container and forceps must be scrubbed and boiled daily and at any time when they become contaminated.

If boiling is the only method available there must be rigid adherence to the following instructions.

The steriliser must be spotlessly clean and filled with sufficient clean water to cover the articles. Timing starts when the water boils and stays boiling for five full minutes and during this time nothing extra must be added. The articles, such as bowls or instruments, must have been scrubbed clean with soap and water and all blood or pus removed before being put into the steriliser.

Glassware should be put into cool water and brought to the boil as it is easily broken by hot water. When sterilising instruments 2% Sodium Carbonate may be added to the water as it raises the boiling point of water and diminishes the rusting of metal. On completion of the 5 minute boiling time instruments should be removed and placed in a sterile covered container and used immediately.

Autoclaving

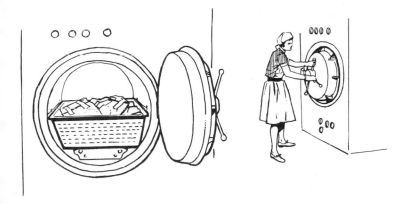

This method of sterilisation uses steam under pressure for a specified length of time and then dries the articles. Most articles including dressings, instruments, needles and glassware can be autoclaved and are packed in packages or boxes on which there is a sensitive strip which changes colour during the process to indicate

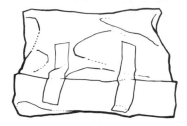 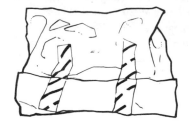

that sterilisation has taken place. All articles must be clean prior to autoclaving. This is an efficient method, as, properly used, it kills micro-organisms and spores.

Dry Heat

This method uses a hot air oven and is an efficient method of killing micro-organisms and spores on glassware and syringes.

Gamma Radiation

This method is one used widely by the large commercial concerns supplying in bulk to hospitals to sterilise articles such as disposable syringes, catheters and tubes.

Chemicals

Chemicals are not efficient in sterilising articles contaminated by spore bearing organisms. Formalin vapour and formalin solution are exceptions and can be used to sterilise articles which would be destroyed by heat.

Some chemicals can destroy non-sporing micro-organisms, for example chlorhexidine or chlorhexidine combined with cetrimide. A nurse should always check carefully on the strength of a solution to make sure that it is at the correct strength for sterilising any particular article.

Sterile Articles in Hospital

Many hospitals now have Central Sterile Supply Departments which clean and sterilise articles and prepare them in packs for individual procedures. As well as, or instead of these, hospitals also make use of equipment prepared and sterilised by commercial concerns.

When these items arrive at the ward and before use it is the nurse's duty to check that the articles are sterile by reference to the control strip, to see that they have not been contaminated by moisture and that the packet is still sealed.

Hands, unlike many other articles, cannot be sterilised so the nurse must remember that, when removing sterile articles from a pack, she must make sure that she does not contaminate the inside of the pack by touching it with her hands.

3
Preparation for Surgery

The preparation required before surgery will vary depending on the type of operation involved. These particular operations will be dealt with in later chapters but there are several features common to all operations and these will be dealt with as follows. The aim in preparing a patient for surgery is, to have him in as fit a condition for operation as is possible, to ensure his safety and to prevent complications occurring.

Admission

Prior to admission the patient may be seen by his General Practitioner and hospitalisation arranged through an Out-patient Clinic or by a Specialist calling at the patient's home. Within a family unit, admission to hospital is not, as it is to the nurse, an every day occurrence, so it is often accompanied by anxiety or perhaps even fear. The nurse can help by remembering this and by caring for her patient as she herself would wish to be treated. It is bad practice and the height of bad manners to refer to a patient as "a case", "bed number 10" or "the appendix". Except in emergencies, patients should be given adequate warning of admission to allow them time to organise personal affairs, such as arranging a replacement at work or for someone to look after a family or aged relative. In emergencies the nurse has a responsibility to see that relatives are informed of admission if they are unaware of its occurrence.

Ideally a patient should be admitted a few days prior to surgery, but if this is not possible more investigations will be carried out on an Out-patient basis. On admission, fear and anxiety may be relieved if the patient has an opportunity to express these to the doctor or nurse. They in turn can explain and reassure or can call upon the services of a senior member of nursing or medical staff to deal with them, or upon the clergy or medical social worker if the problem is one more relevant to their sphere of work. A junior nurse should not attempt to explain something which she does not understand to a patient or his relatives. If she finds herself in this position she should say that she will refer the problem to a senior person who can deal with it for the patient. Adequate information to patient and relatives can often allay anxiety. Some hospitals issue booklets of information. These have been found to be very helpful. Such items as visiting arrangements, articles for the patient to bring in on admission, how to obtain information and from whom, what telephone may be used, the services available to the patient and relatives while the person is in the hospital, travel routes to the hospital, and perhaps also some information about uniforms worn by the various grades of staff. Family anxiety can be communicated to the patient, so explanations and reassurance should be given to them providing the patient has no objection to information regarding his condition being divulged to his relatives. As an individual, the nurse can establish confidence by a clean, smart appearance and efficient, but kindly manner. An unkempt appearance or abrupt manner undermines the patient's confidence and can deter him from asking for information or giving some, which might influence his care or treatment.

Rest, both physical and mental, prepares a person to withstand the strain of operation. To ensure this, nurse should set about the tasks required for the patient's preparation before operation in a calm, efficient manner, and the doctor or the anaesthetist may order a sedative at night to ensure that the patient sleeps well prior to his operation. Although it is the doctor's responsibility to examine the patient clinically and take a history of his illness, the nurse can do much to assist by careful observations of the patient on admission and during his subsequent stay in hospital. During the clinical examination a nurse may assist, and her responsibility is to make sure that the patient has her moral support, is not unnecessarily exposed, and is kept as comfortable as possible throughout the examination. She may also be required to prepare equipment for examinations (e.g. via the vagina or rectum).

4
Methods of Diagnosis

Tests and investigations may be carried out prior to surgery either as an in-patient or out-patient. Many are the doctor's responsibility, such as ordering blood tests, electrocardiograms and x-rays, but the nurse may require to prepare the patient for these tests. Some tests may be long and tedious, and adequate explanation of these and an indication of when results are expected should be given to patients and relatives as this may relieve anxiety and inspire confidence. Investigations for which the nurse is often responsible are urine testing and weighing of patients. Accuracy in urine testing pre-operatively is most important as the results may indicate kidney disease or even diabetes mellitus, in which case there would be special arrangements for anaesthesia. When weighing a patient at regular intervals he must be dressed in the same weight of clothing on each occasion otherwise discrepancies in recordings will occur.

All results of urine testing or weighing must be written down and referred to the person in charge of the ward.

Radiological Examination

X-ray examinations are common aids to diagnosis and are of several types, but from the nurse's point of view there is some basic preparation for any x-ray examination.

The patient should be dressed in a plain gown, generally cotton, without buttons or metal fastenings. The patient should have an explanation of the x-ray and be instructed on what, if anything, he will be expected to do when being x-rayed. An opportunity to use a bedpan or to visit the toilet should be given. If the patient is being x-rayed in the ward, the nurse should assist in the positioning of the patient. If the examination is held in the x-ray department the patient should be taken by trolley or chair. He should be warmly clad in bed socks, slippers and dressing gown and sufficient blankets to keep him comfortable during his journey. Any previous films should be sent or made available with the patient. Nurse should always remember to keep or to order a late meal if the examination intrudes on meal times. If the patient's condition allows, he should be allowed to move around prior to x-ray examination as this helps to discourage the collection of gas in the intestinal tract. This will therefore make reading of the x-rays an easier task for the Radiologist.

Types of X-ray

Direct x-ray photograph or straight x-ray of a part may show up, perhaps gall stones, a swallowed foreign body or may show the presence of a tumour or disease. At other times to outline a part of the body which would not show up with an ordinary straight x-ray, it is necessary for a dye or a radio-opaque substance to be introduced into the body. Barium sulphate may be used to outline the alimentary tract. When given orally for a barium swallow, it outlines the oesophagus, for a barium meal, it outlines the stomach and the first part of the small intestine. Barium can also be given as an enema and will outline the rectum and large bowel.

The gall bladder can be outlined by giving a dye in tablet form or intravenously. This is called a cholecystogram. A dye can outline the biliary ducts producing a cholangiogram.

Similarly, dye can be introduced intravenously and x-rays taken of kidneys (intravenous pyelogram), or introduced directly into the bladder to outline this structure (cystogram). Special preparation may be required for these more complex x-ray investigations and each individual hospital has its own particular ideas on preparation. Suggested preparation will be found in the appendix.

Endoscopic Examination

If there is a blemish on the skin, the doctor can see this without much trouble, but he may wish to look at a more inaccessible part of the patient, for example, the inside of the oesophagus or rectum, and to do this he will require to introduce a hollow tube into the organ. Names given to these examinations are as follows

1. Examination of the oesophagus — oesophagoscopy

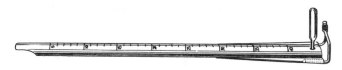

Oesophagoscope

2. Examination of the stomach — gastroscopy or fibroscopy

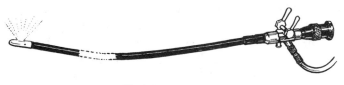

Gastroscope

3. Examination of the lower bowel — sigmoidoscopy

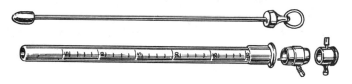

Sigmoidoscope

4. Examination of the rectum — proctoscopy

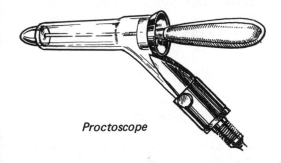

Proctoscope

5. Examination of the air passages — bronchoscopy

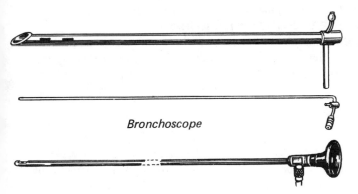

Bronchoscope

6. Examination of the bladder — cystoscopy

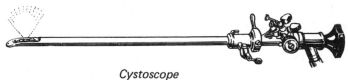

Cystoscope

hese examinations may require a local or general anaesthetic.

Biopsy

To confirm or make a diagnosis, the doctor has sometimes to remove a piece of tissue under local or general anaesthetic so that the pathologist can decide if it is diseased or not. This procedure is called taking a biopsy.

Laboratory Examination

Doctor may send any discharges, secretions or excretions, for example, pus, gastric juice or faeces to a laboratory to be examined. These are often collected by the nurse.

Doctor may also wish blood to be examined and this he collects himself and despatches to the laboratory for assessment or to the blood transfusion department for blood grouping and cross matching, so that blood can be available for a patient if he requires this as part of treatment or in the post-operative phase.

The patient must be in the best possible health before anaesthesia. Doctor will order treatment for any anaemia, sepsis or dehydration. The diet should, if possible, be rich in vitamins and proteins. It may be adjusted if the patient's illness requires (e.g. a low residue diet or a fluid diet).

Drugs to treat disease or as a preparation for example of the bowel may be given prior to surgery. These are ordered by doctor and the nurse must take great care to check adequately that the correct drug is given to the correct patient in the correct dosage, at the correct time by the correct route. After operation the patient will require to perform breathing exercises to prevent chest complications. These exercises should be taught and practiced prior to operation. The physiotherapist is unable to spend much time with the patient so he relies on the nurse for help, continuity, and encouragement with these. Lack of knowledge of pre- and post-operative care may give rise to tensions within the patient. The nurse must therefore explain to the patient about having to stay in bed for a day or so after operation, necessitating the use of urinals and/ or bed pans and patients should have an opportunity to use these prior to theatre so that the experience after operation is not too strange for them. The possible presence of intravenous fluids, catheter drainage or splints should be mentioned so that the patient and relatives are not alarmed unnecessarily at a later date. If the position of a patient's bed has to be changed to allow for the use of oxygen or suction or for convenience of observation post-operatively, the patient should have this explanation prior to going to theatre.

If the patient is to have major changes in his way of life after operation (e.g. a colostomy or an amputation), nurse must help to explain these to the patient, but the main explanation and the responsibility for giving it belongs to the doctor or surgeon. The anaesthetist will see the patient prior to theatre and explain the induction of anaesthesia, which may be by injection or inhalation. It is also explained that a period of fasting is required so that the stomach contents are not inhaled during the anaesthetic. Smoking should be avoided as it predisposes to post operative chest infections.

An important part of preparation is the signing of "Consent for Treatment and Operation Form". It may be the nurse's duty to obtain the patient's signature for this, but explanation regarding the nature of operation is given by the doctor, or surgeon.

CONSENT BY OR ON BEHALF OF PATIENT

I ....

of ....

consent to the submission of *myself ....

to the operation of ....

the nature and purpose of which have been explained to me.

I also consent to such further or alternative operative measures as may be found necessary during the course of such operation and to the administration of a local or other anaesthetic for any of the foregoing purposes.

I understand that an assurance has not been given that the operation will be performed by any specified surgeon.

                                                            *Patient

Date ....Signed..................................... Parent
                                                            Guardian

*Delete where inapplicable.

I confirm that I have explained to the patient the nature and purpose of the proposed operation.

Date ....Signed....................................(Medical Practitioner)

REFUSAL OF TREATMENT

                                               Hospital No.

I..

of..

hereby declare that I am leaving *(or taking .... away from)

the ....Hospital at my own desire and contrary to the advice of the medical staff.   I have had the risks of so doing explained to me, and I accept full responsibility for my action.

                                  Signature ....

Date.....................   Witness..............................

* Delete whichever is inapplicable.

5
Pre-operative Nursing Care

The care given immediately pre-operatively is as follows, but the nurse must realise that in emergency situations all of this may not be completed, but as much as possible should be attempted. The points which have already been mentioned in preparation for surgery require to be explained to the patient and the patient reassured so that his co-operation is gained and he is not unnecessarily concerned.

Stomach and Bowel

The stomach is emptied prior to anaesthetic so that during it, inhalation of stomach contents does not occur, and after operation the risk of vomiting is reduced. There are a few ways in which this can be achieved. The patient may be starved for approximately four to six hours pre-operatively, but if there is a danger that, by doing this, the patient may become dehydrated, doctor may start an intravenous infusion to allow the patient to have adequate fluids via another route rather than the gastro-intestinal route.

Another method of emptying the stomach is by aspirating the contents and this is done by means of a naso-gastric tube being passed into the stomach, a syringe or suction machine being attached to the end and the contents withdrawn.

A third possibility is washing out the stomach by means of a gastric lavage and this should be done, for example, when a patient has a pyloric stenosis. No matter which way is used the patient should be given a clear explanation for each situation and any food, fluid, sweets or fruit should be carefully stored out of reach of the patient so that he does not inadvertently take anything in the immediate pre-operative phase.

The bowel may or may not be given special preparation. If required, an aperient, suppositories, enema or lavage may be used. The bowel preparation may last over a few days if the bowel is the site of operation or only the night prior to or on the morning of the operation prior to other types of surgery. Whichever method is used will depend on what operation the patient is having performed, but peristalsis should always be allowed to subside prior to operation after any of these treatments.

Bladder

The bladder should be emptied prior to the anaesthetic. This can be done by a patient passing urine in the normal way before going to theatre or on infrequent occasions catheterisation may be required. If the patient does not pass urine, theatre should be informed in writing as a full bladder is easily punctured during abdominal or pelvic surgery. The patient should be allowed to empty his bladder prior to the administration of the pre-medication (pre-anaesthetic drug). There is then less chance of the patient being unable to use a urinal or bed pan properly, or of him falling out of bed, due to the drug making him drowsy.

Cleanliness of Skin and Nails

The area of, and the area surrounding, the operation site is generally shaved. It is easier to shave the axilla or pubic area if the hair is cut short prior to shaving. Shaving should be done with a clean razor and a new blade. Great care is taken to ensure that the skin is not cut. Abrasions and cuts allow entrance of infection. The razor, if nondisposable, should be sterilised after use. The skin should be thoroughly washed after shaving and special attention given to skin folds such as the groins. The umbilicus may very well require special attention. If it is full of skin debris, olive oil soaks should be applied on admission so that by the time operation is due the umbilicus will be clean and less likely to harbour micro-organisms. The surgeon may give special instructions regarding the use of antiseptic solutions, but these would be prescribed for the individual patient. A bath should be given on the day before operation, except in an emergency when, if possible and his condition allows, the patient would be bathed prior to operation. Cleanliness of skin and umbilicus must be checked.

If a long post-operative phase is envisaged and the patient is fit enough, a shampoo may be given prior to operation. If the patient is menstruating a clean sanitary towel should be applied prior to going to theatre, and the theatre sister must be informed of its presence. Normally internal sanitary towels are not left in position before the patient goes to theatre.

Any nail varnish or facial make-up must be removed before the patient goes to theatre as the anaesthetist will be observing the state of the circulation by looking at the colour of the patient's nails and face, and if these are highly or even faintly coloured artificially his observations may be misleading. The patient's nails must be clean and short to prevent damage to himself or to the staff while he is being moved from bed to trolley or trolley to theatre table. The patient's mouth must be clean before leaving for theatre as any debris could be introduced into the lungs when the endotracheal tube is being passed.

Rest and Sleep

To ensure that the patient is rested prior to operation the ward in which he is nursed must be well ventilated, without draughts, be warm enough to be comfortable and the bustle and noise of the ward kept to a minimum. The evening before operation the doctor generally orders night sedation for the patient if he thinks that this will be necessary to ensure a good night's rest.

Premedication

Prior to the patient going to theatre the anaesthetist orders a drug called a premedication or pre-anaesthetic drug to be given. He may order the sedation at the same time as he does this. The premedication is a drug given to the patient to reduce the amount of secretions from the various glands in the mouth and thus cut down the risk of secretions filling the lungs during operation. It is also given to calm the patient prior to operation. It is essential that the correct drug is given at the correct time, at the correct site, by the correct method of injection ordered. If there is unavoidable delay, it is essential that the anaesthetist is informed of this so that he may judge the effect of the premedication by the length of time from which it was given. If, however, the anaesthetist feels that with the change in time the premedication will not be useful he may give the drug intravenously in the anaesthetic room. At no time should a nurse attempt to conceal any delay in giving premedication, and the time at which it is given must be correctly stated on the anaesthetic sheet. Any other practice may be harmful to the patient. When this premedication is being given the nurse must explain its purpose to the patient as otherwise he may not understand why his mouth is so dry and why he feels drowsy.

Dress for Theatre

It is important to plan the preparation of the patient for theatre in a careful fashion so that the patient is not lying dressed ready for theatre for long periods of time. Normally the gown worn for theatre is a simple cotton or terry-towelling gown fastening with tapes at the back. The patient's hair must be covered by a cap which may be of the paper disposable variety or merely a triangle of calico. Any hair ornaments or metal clips which the patient has in his or her hair must be removed prior to covering it. It is easier if the long hair is plaited prior to covering it with the cap. Any artificial aids must be removed before the patient leaves the ward for theatre. Dentures should be removed and if they are not already clean they should be cleaned and stored in a labelled container, either inside the patient's locker or in a locked cupboard used specifically for this purpose. Nurses must not forget that some patients have artificial limbs or a prosthesis such as a breast or an eye. These must be removed, labelled, and stored in a safe place so that no inconvenience is caused to the patient on his return from theatre.

Any rings which the patient may be wearing should be taken off, labelled, and stored, and they should be cared for as a nurse would normally care for patients valuables. If the patient has a wedding ring and wishes to leave this on, this is generally acceptable provided the ring is covered with adhesive tape. The exceptions to such an arrangement would be if the patient's operation was one on the hand or wrist where the nurse would expect some swelling to occur post operatively and therefore it is best if the ring is removed.

Recordings and Observations

The temperature, pulse and respirations must be observed on the day of operation and the nurse must report any rise or any abnormality in any of these three recordings. Many nurses are requested to record the patient's blood pressure prior to operation as this will give a guide as to whether the blood pressure recorded post operatively is normal for this patient or not. If the patient has any signs of fever, such as rise in temperature or sore throat or dyspnoea this must be reported as it may mean cancellation of operation. Most patients are anxious prior to theatre, but any undue anxiety should be reported to the person in charge of the ward.

Check Documents, Equipment and Patient

As well as checking the permission for operation and treatment form on admission of the patient, this must also be checked prior to the patient leaving the ward for theatre. The nurse must also check that the identity of the patient is in no doubt and that bracelets of identification are in position. If these are not used an adhesive label or a tie on label should be attached to the patient's wrist, giving details of name, hospital and ward number. The nurse should check that she knows what operation the patient is expected to have and if it is involving a limb she should know which limb. Doctor may mark the site before operation to prevent any chance of error. Any x-rays which the patient has had taken prior to theatre should accompany him as should also his case sheet and any other details required by the surgeon in theatre. Any written notes to the theatre sister or to the anaesthetist regarding any upset in preparation should also accompany the patient.

Transporting the Patient

The patient's position on the trolley should be carefully checked. The canvas with its cover of a sheet should be under the patient and the patient's head must rest on a pillow on this canvas to ensure that the head and neck are not jerked backwards when the patient is unconscious and being placed on the theatre table. When helping or lifting a patient from the bed to the trolley it is important that the nurses position the limbs of the patient carefully so that they are not damaged by being caught between bed and trolley. During transportation to theatre, the nurse, generally the ward nurse, accompanies the patient and she should have all the information required by the theatre personnel in her keeping during this time. She should also be there to give the patient moral support and often stays until the patient's anaesthetic has been induced.

Prepare Bed and Equipment for Return

Once the patient has left the ward for theatre his bed should be stripped and remade with fresh linen so that, should the operation take a shorter time than expected, the bed will be ready to receive the patient. Any special equipment, charts, suction or oxygen and any drainage bags should be ready as soon as possible after the patient has gone to theatre for the same reason.

Relatives

It is important that the hospital has some means of contacting relatives when the patient is going to theatre so that they can be informed of any delay or cancellation. The relatives should be given a time to 'phone the ward for information regarding the patient's post-operative condition.

6
Post-operative Nursing Care

The aim in post operative nursing care is
1. To observe the patient
2. To prevent complications
3. To relieve pain
4. To return the patient to normality as soon as possible.

This will be considered in two sections
a) immediate post operative care
b) the phase of convalescence.

Post operative care after special operations will be dealt with in the appropriate section. The purpose of this section is to deal with the general care required after any operation.

Immediate Post-operative Care

Preparation for Return

As already mentioned, as soon as the patient has left the ward, the nurse should prepare for his return as the operation may be short or take less time than was originally envisaged. The patient's bed should be made up with fresh linen and the upper bed clothes should

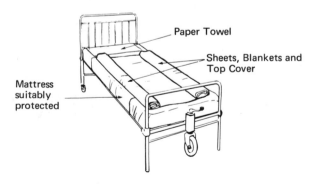

Paper Towel

Sheets, Blankets and Top Cover

Mattress suitably protected

be arranged in a pack so that they can be easily moved when the patient returns from the theatre.

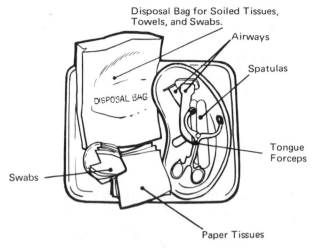

Disposal Bag for Soiled Tissues, Towels, and Swabs.

Airways

Spatulas

DISPOSAL BAG

Tongue Forceps

Swabs

Paper Tissues

On bedtable or locker a tray containing a mouth gag, airway, tongue forceps and tongue depressors should always be ready so that the nurse can cope on the patient's return if he should obstruct his airway with his tongue. A suction machine, tubing and a selection of catheters should also be available in case the airway becomes blocked with secretions. Nurse must check any connections to be used and make sure that they will fit the available catheter and tubing. An oxygen supply, tubing and appropriate mask should be ready, should the patient require oxygen post operatively. Charts for post operative recordings should be named and made ready and these may include blood pressure, temperature, pulse, respiratory rate charts, fluid balance charts and the equipment required for these records such as thermometer, a watch with a second hand, a sphygmomanometer and stethescope. If the bed does not have inbuilt elevating controls, a bed elevator should be available in case the patient is shocked. Nurse will have, in most circumstances, some indication prior to theatre, what operation is likely to be performed, therefore special drainage bags or bottles, wound or gastro-intestinal suction, intravenous infusion stand or any other equipment which she expects will be needed should be checked and made ready for the patient's return.

Transportation from Theatre

After operation the patient may be looked after in a recovery room or be returned to the ward from which he came. He may return in his own bed or on a trolley, but no matter which way he goes, he should be accompanied by a porter and nurse and if he

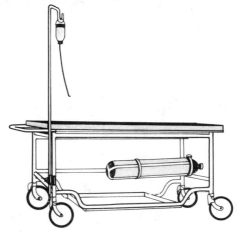

Theatre trolley

is still unconscious it is nurse's responsibility to ensure that a clear airway is maintained. The trolley or bed should therefore be equipped with oxygen and mask, and the nurse should support the patient's jaw to help keep his airway clear. It is important that if he is lifted into bed that his arms and legs are not damaged by either hanging over the side of the trolley or being caught between the trolley and the bed. Care should be taken that infusions or drains are not displaced when the patient is moved. Gentle handling of the patient is essential if he is not to become even more shocked after operation.

There will be a written post-operative instruction sheet supplied by the surgeon or doctor in theatre, and this should be returned to the ward with the patient's case sheet and x-rays.

Positioning in Bed

When placed in bed the first essential is to maintain a clear airway, and this can be done either by placing the patient in a semi prone position or if this is not suitable to the type of operation performed the patient may lie in the lateral position. Inhalation of secretions or

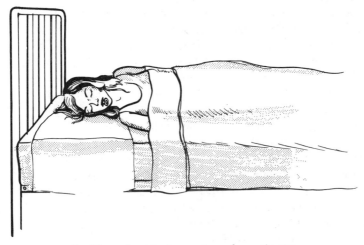

Position of patient on return from theatre

vomiting is less likely to occur if these positions are adopted while the patient is unconscious. In most instances the anaesthetist leaves an artificial airway in position and the patient should remove this himself or be allowed to spit it out. It must never be forced from his mouth by the nurse. The positioning of the patient, as well as allowing for a clear airway, should allow for the observation of the wound, any drainage and also for any recordings which are to be made. The patient should also be as comfortable as is possible.

While the patient is unconscious he must never be left unattended. The patient must be carefully observed both during the initial post operative phase while he is unconscious and on regaining consciousness.

Observations

One of the complications which can occur postoperatively is asphyxia (suffocation). To prevent this occurrence the nurse must always observe that, and ensure that, the patient's airway is clear. The patient's colour will also give some indication if the oxygen is entering the lungs and getting into the blood stream. A bluish tinge round the patient's lips, nose or ear lobes would indicate that this was not happening.

The pulse rate should be recorded at regular intervals as a rise in pulse rate may indicate that the patient is bleeding. A further aid to observing the amount of shock or bleeding is the recording of the blood pressure. If this should fall below 100 mm.Hg. (millimetres of mercury) systolic pressure, doctor should be informed.

Note should also be made of the patient's temperature and respiration. A rise in temperature and difficulty in breathing may indicate that the patient is developing a chest infection.

Some pain is to be expected after the effects of anaesthesia have worn off. Doctor will have ordered a drug to relieve this and it should be given when the patient shows signs of discomfort or pain.

Vomiting may occur post-operatively and the nurse should observe the appearance and the quantity and should note this on the fluid balance chart. If the patient is having naso-gastric suction the pressure should not rise above 5 cm.Hg. on the suction machine. The contents of the stomach which are aspirated should be observed and the quantity noted on the fluid balance chart.

The nurse should observe when the patient passes urine but should not expect this immediately on return from theatre as the patient may have had a restricted fluid intake prior to theatre and one would not therefore expect his bladder to be full. However, if the patient does not empty his bladder within 8 hours of operation, the matter would be reported to sister or the doctor. Nurse should encourage the patient to empty his bladder by providing the privacy which the patient would desire. The added stimulus of the sound of running water helps!! Position him in a comfortable way for voiding and make sure that the urinal or bedpan is warm and dry.

As a result of operation there is occasionally some upset in the movement of the gastro-intestinal tract and the patient should therefore be observed to see if he passes any flatus and this reported to sister. If gas collects in the bowel and the abdomen becomes distended, it may be relieved by passing a flatus tube into the rectum and allowing the gas to escape.

The patient's wound should be observed for any staining, either with serous fluid, blood, or any other discharge and any odour should be noted. If a drain is in position some discharge would be expected from the wound, otherwise there should be little or no staining from the wound.

These are the main observations which would be carried out in the initial post operative period. The frequency would depend on how shocked the patient was after operation. The frequency of observations would be decreased when the patient's condition improved and on return to consciousness.

The patient's head and shoulders should gradually be elevated on pillows only after consciousness is regained. He should be reassured about his operation and visited by the surgeon. The patient's mouth will be dry since he was probably given a drug prior to theatre to reduce the amount of secretions in his mouth. The patient's fluid intake was also probably restricted and as the patient has perhaps had an inhaled anaesthetic this will also make his mouth dry. It should therefore be carefully swabbed clean or if the patient's condition allows he should have a mouth wash. The patient's general hygiene should be attended to but in the initial stages after operation sponging of the hands and the face will be sufficient, and if at the same time his gown is changed and his position checked to make sure that he is comfortable it will allow him to feel more settled and happier after coming back from theatre. Physiotherapy of the appropriate type should be instigated as soon as possible after operation, providing this is in accordance with the doctor's orders.

Continued Care

As the patient's condition improves and to prevent complications occurring, it is desirable to get the patient moving, first of all in bed and eventually to sit up and walk. Patients should never be left on their own when they get up to walk for the first time and should always be accompanied the first time they go to the toilet after operation so that they do not fall. When the patient is allowed up to sit he must only be up for the time stated by doctor as any more than this may be tiring and harmful to the patient. The patient must be helped in and

57

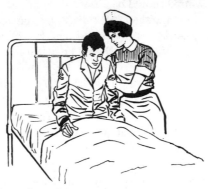

out of bed until fit and confident to manage on his own.

The patient may require drugs post-operatively, such as anti-biotics, or iron tablets and many surgeons like their patients to have additional vitamins given after operation to promote healing of the wound. The patient's diet will be adapted depending on his needs. This may initially be given by the intravenous route and gradually introduced as an oral administration of diet in the fluid form and then on to perhaps a light or an ordinary diet. Post operative aperients may be given if the bowel does not move normally. These must be ordered by doctor. The patient's wound would be observed and care given to it. This is dealt with in more detail in the section on wound care.

The patient must be rehabilitated and educated from the moment he is admitted. According to his age and intelligence, he should have an explanation of his disease and if it is permissible his relatives should also have a similar explanation.

7
Complications

Prevention of some Common Complications following Operation

Apart from the complications such as asphyxia and urine retention which have already been mentioned there are other complications which may occur in the post operative period. The most common ones are pain, gastro-intestinal upsets, haemorrhage, sepsis, deep venous thrombosis, chest infections and paralytic ileus.

Patients may try to bear discomfort or pain without complaint so the nurse must observe any restlessness, make sure that the bed is warm and the patient's position is comfortable. If these measures are inadequate analgesics may be given by doctor once the cause of the discomfort or pain has been ascertained.

The patient may vomit after operation and, as already mentioned, this should be reported. Nurse must, however, remember to remove the soiled sickness basin and supply a clean one so nausea is not induced by the smell or sight of vomitus. The patient should be handled gently and kindly, any soiling of the skin or bed linen cleaned and the patient's mouth should be swabbed or he should be given a mouth wash. Flatulence may be relieved by positioning the patient so that gas can be expelled from the stomach. The administration of warm drinks, if allowed, is often helpful.

Constipation may occur post-operatively. Encouraging the patient to take fluids and his diet, to move round in bed; providing a bedpan or commode in privacy when required may help prevent its occurrence.

Haemorrhage may occur within the first 24 hours of operation or perhaps during the first post operative week. The patients should be observed carefully during this time. If haemorrhage occurs, doctor must be informed, the nurse must apply a firm sterile dressing over the bleeding site and reassure the patient.

Sepsis may occur and will be mentioned in the section on wound care.

Deep Venous Thrombosis (clotting in the deep veins of the

leg or pelvis) may occur in the post-operative period. Nurse should note any rise in temperature and any pain or tenderness in the leg and report this. This may be prevented by encouraging the patient to move freely in bed and being careful that there is no undue pressure on the patient's legs while in bed. A piece of this thrombus may become dislodged and travel in the blood stream and block one of the blood vessels in the lungs. This would be called a Pulmonary Embolus. If it was large it could be fatal.

Chest complications such as pneumonia may occur and the nurse can help to prevent these by encouraging the patient to do deep breathing exercises and cough at regular intervals. While doing so the patient should be taught to support his wound so that pain and discomfort is reduced. The nurse should report any pain or difficulty in breathing which the patient may experience as this may be a sign of complications in the chest.

A paralytic ileus is paralysis of a portion of the bowel and may follow an operation where there has been a lot of handling of the bowel. The nurse should observe the patient for vomiting and abdominal discomfort and distention. The patient will not pass flatus or faeces. If these signs and symptoms are noted nurse must report them immediately.

8
Dismissal

Written instructions must always be given to the patient or his relatives on dismissal. In the excitement of going home it is easy to forget instructions which one is given, therefore these must be written down. Instructions should be given on the diet which has to be followed, the amount of activity allowed, any drugs which have to be taken, any dressings or baths which have to be done or taken and the patient should be informed if and when he ought to return to the clinic. If his appointment is to be sent to him by post the patient should be informed of this. If any special equipment is required for the patient's care this should be ordered at an early stage of his illness. If the patient is discharged to his own home, doctor informs his General Practitioner and, if care from the District Nurse is required this should be arranged before dismissal.

If the patient is discharged for convalescence to another hospital it is of the utmost importance that the patient's relatives are fully informed of these arrangements so that they can be given information regarding visiting hours and travelling instructions before their relative leaves the ward. If this practice is not followed relatives can be very distressed at visiting hour by finding the bed in which their next of kin was being nursed empty, so it is of the greatest importance that they know of any transfer to another ward or discharge to another hospital which may have been arranged.

Sometimes the results of a surgical operation are not successful and the patient is very ill and eventually dies. The bed is usually screened at this stage.

After death has been certified by doctor, the nurse should remove any drains or dressings and cover the wound with a fresh covering. Unless a mortician is available the nurse should wash the patient, comb the hair into its usual style and dress the patient in a shroud or clothing recommended by the particular hospital. This should be done quickly, efficiently and quietly as it can be distressing to the other patients. An identification card or bracelet should be attached to the patient's body. The body should be left in a clean bed and all equipment should be removed from the bedside. A porter will be called to convey the body to the mortuary.

During the phase of the patient's illness prior to his death the nurse must give the patient all the support and care necessary. The relatives and patient may wish to see the medical social worker or spiritual advisor and assistance should be given by the nurse. Even when it is expected, the death of a loved one is a shattering blow. A nurse must realise this fully and, without becoming emotionally involved, by her presence and practical help assist the bereaved relatives as much as possible. A cup of tea at a time like this may be of little practical use, but is often acceptable as it illustrates the concern of the staff for the relatives. A calm, understanding, kindly manner is essential in the nurse. There is no place for the brash, brisk or unfeeling attitude which adds further distress to relatives.

After the formalities are dealt with it is the nurse's responsibility to see that the relatives are in a fit state to journey home. If a post mortem examination is required the issue of a death certificate may be delayed. Doctor will make arrangements with the relatives regarding the collection of the certificate.

9
Dressings

The skin acts as a barrier to invasion of the body by micro-organisms and if it is broken infection is much more likely to occur.

After operation the patient is left with a wound made by sterile instruments and sewn or sealed by sterile materials. In caring for this wound the aim is to keep the wound free from infection. To do this the wound is rarely disturbed until it is time for sutures or clips to be removed. Exceptions to this are if the patient's pulse rate or temperature rise, if pain or undue discomfort is experienced over the site of the wound or if there is any inflammation, swelling or discharge, in which case the wound would be inspected and the dressings renewed as there is a possibility that it has become infected.

Different types of wounds require individual management but the basic principles are the same no matter what has to be done.

As mentioned in a previous chapter, infection travels via the air, dust, soiled articles, contaminated hands and clothing, so that to avoid contamination of a wound an aseptic technique must be used. This means that the equipment and dressings used must be sterile and that the wound must not be touched by any article which is not sterile, and particularly it must not be touched by the hands.

Ideally, for one hour prior to dressings commencing in the ward the activity in the ward should be at a minimum and these conditions should prevail until the dressings are completed. Bed making, toilet rounds, domestic tasks can stir up dust containing micro-organisms. An alternative arrangement is that dressings can be carried out in a special room set aside for that purpose. If several dressings have to be carried out the cleanest and newest wound should be attended to first and gradually the dressings which are then done become more and more of a contaminated type. The dresser and her assistant must have a high standard of personal hygiene and be neatly dressed. Hair should be well controlled as it can carry infection and dust from it can be introduced into a wound. Anyone who has any sepsis or respiratory infection should not be in a surgical ward let alone be taking part in ward dressings.

Some authorities advocate the use of masks to prevent the spread of micro-organisms from the nurse to the patient. Other authorities do not. If masks are worn they should be put on carefully making

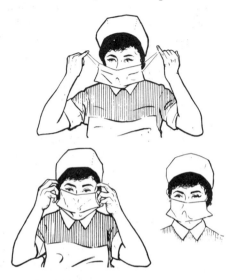

sure that the nose and mouth are covered. Once in position they must not be touched till it is time for removal and they are then removed by loosening the tapes from behind the ears and dropping the soiled mask, touching only the tapes, into a pedal bin or container for the purpose. Masks should never be worn longer than 20 minutes and should always be changed on completion of each dressing. Most masks nowadays are of the disposable variety. If masks are not worn conversation should be severely restricted during the procedure.

The nurse must make sure that her nails are clean prior to doing dressings and that here hands are washed prior to setting up, prior to doing the actual dressing, and on completion of the procedure. To wash her hands the nurse should use a wash basin with taps which can be turned off using the elbows. A bacteriostatic soap or solution should be used to wash the hands to above the level of the wrists. This lather should then be rinsed off thoroughly and the hands dried very carefully on a clean towel. If the hands are left wet the skin may become hacked and may harbour micro-organisms. By washing and drying her hands carefully a nurse can rid her skin of many of the micro-organisms which may be on it but they will never become sterile therefore they should never be in contact with the patient's wound as this can lead to contamination and possible infection of it.

The trolley which is used should be a double shelved trolley and one which is kept for the purpose. It is washed using soap or an antiseptic solution and dried before and after each dressing using a disposable cloth or paper towel.

The solutions used for cleaning a wound should be uncontaminated by micro-organisms and be in clearly labelled bottles. The dressings should be contained in individual packets and may have the instruments in with them or in a separate packet or tube. The packet of the most useful size for the dressing should be selected and checked to see that it is sterile and has neither a broken seal nor is contaminated by any dampness. Likewise the instrument tube or packet.

The dressing may be secured by a bandage or some type of adhesive and clean scissors must be available for cutting the latter.

Throughout the procedure neither the patient, the dresser, nor her assistant should touch with their hands the wound, any dressing towel or inner dressings, whether soiled or sterile.

The patient should have an opportunity to visit the toilet or use a bedpan a short time prior to the procedure to prevent interruption of the dressing. Disposal bags are required for soiled articles and these must always be closed before the nurse removes her trolley from the bedside.

Outline of Simple Dressings Procedure

The patient's bed should be screened and he should be placed in a position which allows easy access to the wound, but which is also comfortable and any draughts should be excluded. An explanation must be given to the patient and this can be done while he is being settled. If masks are to be worn they should be put on by both nurses before their hands are washed. Hands should be washed using a bacteriostatic soap or solution for one minute, this is rinsed off and the hands carefully dried.

The dresser then washes the trolley with soap or antiseptic solution and dries it carefully. Sterile articles are placed on the top shelf, clean articles are placed on the bottom shelf.

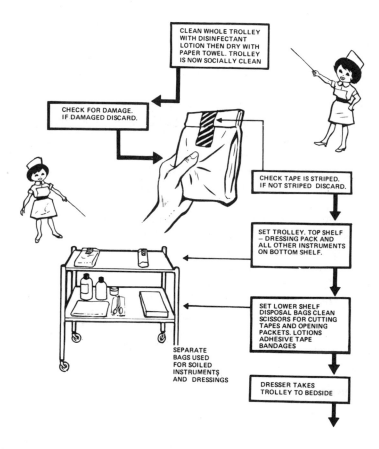

The trolley is then taken to the patient's bedside and the assistant turns back the bedclothes and loosens the patient's clothing.

The dresser opens the dressings packet cutting, if necessary, with clean scissors and drops the contents carefully on to the top shelf.

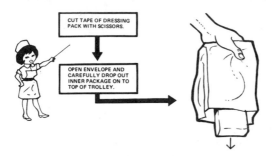

The inside packet is then opened, touching only the outside of the wrapper. If instruments are in a separate packet or tube this is also opened taking great care not to touch either the inside of the container or the contents. The instruments are then dropped in a convenient position on the sterile sheet in which the dressings were wrapped.

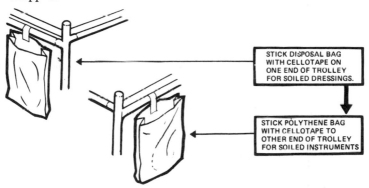

A disposal bag is attached to the side of the trolley using sellotape. If instruments are not disposable, a separate bag is attached for these. This may be a clear polythene bag where the contents can be easily seen and therefore will help to prevent mistaken disposal of non-disposable items.

The dresser loosens the patient's dressing and then washes her hands for one minute and dries them carefully. She must take great care not to touch anything with her hands when returning to the patient's bedside. With a pair of forceps she arranges her dressings material and places a gallipot so that the assistant can fill it with what ever solution the dresser may use.

The solution is checked by the dresser before the assistant pours it into the container. The assistant must be careful to avoid touching any of the sterile articles.

The dresser removes the soiled dressing with a pair of forceps which are then discarded. If while doing the dressing the forceps are to be laid down they should be placed with their points on a sterile swab resting on the sterile sheet on the trolley. A dressings towel is then draped beside the wound using forceps. The wound may or may not require cleaning but should this be required it would be done at this point using swabs held in forceps. The dresser works away from the wound so that micro-organisms are not introduced into it. The wound and the surrounding area are carefully dried.

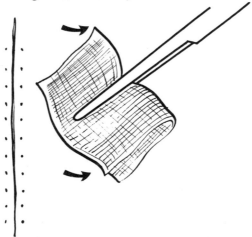

Always swab away from the wound

The dresser than places a fresh dressing over the wound and discards her forceps into the disposal bag. She then unrolls the necessary amount of adhesive which the assistant cuts with clean scissors, this is then secured over the wound. Alternatively a bandage may be used. The dresser then places all disposable items in the disposal bag and seals it. If instruments are in a separate bag this is also sealed.

The dresser and her assistant then make the patient comfortable, remove screens and see that the patient's locker is within easy reach.

Soiled dressings in their bag, are disposed of in a bin which should be outside the ward. If instruments are non disposable these are sent in their bag to the Central Sterile Supply Department. If this is not available they should be soaked in antiseptic solution prior to being scrubbed and packed for autoclaving. The scissors which have been used to cut the packet or tape should be washed between dressings. Solutions and tape are returned to the cupboard and the nurses then remove their masks and drop them into a pedal bin. The trolley is then washed down and the nurses both wash their hands.

It is just as important to prepare everything prior to a dressing and clear up adequately afterwards as it is to follow correctly the procedure of doing a dressing. Immaculate technique is essential to prevent cross infection occurring.

The patient must be instructed not to touch his dressing and no doctor or nurse must attempt to loosen a corner of a dressing to look at the wound. If inspection of a wound is necessary preparations to perform a dressing must be made before the dressing is loosened so that the wound is not contaminated by fingers of nursing or medical personnel and it is not left exposed for an undue length of time.

On completion of the dressing the nurse should report on the condition of the wound to the senior nurse on duty.

10
Care of Wounds and Drains

There are many schools of thought regarding the use of dressings material over surgical wounds. Some authorities like the wound covered only by a thin transparent plastic dressing. If this is of the spray-on variety the nurse must be careful to allow sufficient time for the dressing to dry before settling the patient. Some surgeons feel that since it is best that a wound stays dry, it should be exposed to the atmosphere without covering four or five days after operation. Wounds which involve a weeping or moist surface may have a special non adherent dressing applied, for example, paraffin gauze, and this will save discomfort to the patient and the tearing of fresh healing tissue on its removal. A wound which is infected may have a gauze swab soaked in an antiseptic solution applied over it. A wound with a slough may be treated with soaks of eusol which helps to clean the wound and reduce the odour from it. This substance is only active for a short period of time so the nurse may find that several dressings would be ordered each day on the wound until it is clean.

Each patient, however, is an individual and the nurse must follow carefully any instructions which she is given regarding the care of the wound.

Most dressings which are applied over wounds are made of gauze or non adherent material. This is held in place by a bandage, adhesive plaster or one of the newer types of tape, for example, micro-pore tape.

Bandages which are used may be crepe or cotton open weave, but should mould easily to the part being covered, be applied evenly over it without constricting the circulation and should cover the dressing and also be comfortable for the patient. If adhesive bandage or plaster is used nurse must ascertain that the patient is not allergic to it as some people can develop very uncomfortable or painful rashes on the site of their application. The new types of tape do not seem to cause the same amount of discomfort.

Removal of Sutures and Clips

Sutures or clips are inserted at the time of operation to hold the skin edges together and by so doing encourage the healing process. There are various types of stitching, but when these are being removed the same principle applies. Material which has been lying on the surface of the skin should never be pulled through the underlying tissues as this can introduce infection. The surgeon decides when these sutures should be removed and the length of time will vary, depending on his particular views on the subject and on the site of the wound, for example, wounds of head and neck generally have their sutures left in for two to four days, but the abdominal wall may have the sutures left in it for anything from seven to fourteen days.

To remove sutures a dressings trolley and equipment, as described previously, is necessary, also a pair of forceps capable of grasping the stitch should be available. These may be either dressings or dissecting

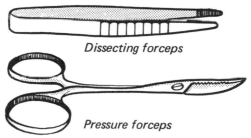

Dissecting forceps

Pressure forceps

forceps and in the case of very tiny sutures being removed mosquito forceps would be required.

To cut the sutures, scissors or stitch cutters may be used. The latter are disposable, which is an obvious advantage.

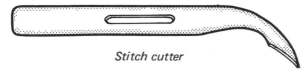

Stitch cutter

Added to their other worries many patients have a fear of suture removal so the nurse should have a firm kindly approach to the patient and should remove sutures without fuss and waste of time.

Interrupted Sutures

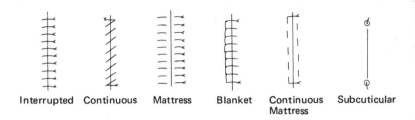

Interrupted   Continuous   Mattress   Blanket   Continuous Mattress   Subcuticular

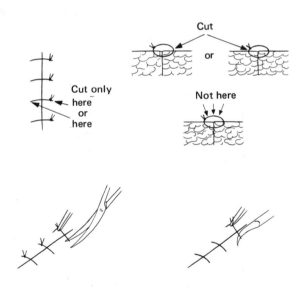

Forceps should be used to lift the thread near the knot. The sutures should be cut where the suture enters the skin. To cut a suture the blades of the scissors or stitch cutters should be laid on the flat of the skin so that the points are not jabbing into the patient and causing unnecessary discomfort. The suture is then drawn out from the tissues.

Removal of Clips

Michel's Clips.

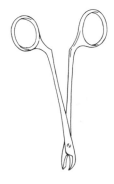

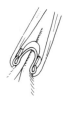

To remove Michel's clips a pair of Michel's clip removing forceps are required and a pair of forceps.

The clip is steadied by the pair of forceps.

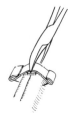

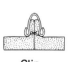

Clip inserted

Method of removal

The point of the Michel's clip removers slipped under the clip.

The forceps are then closed and the pressure on the clip brings the pointed ends out of the skin on either side.

The clip then lifts easily from the surface of the skin.

Profile (Michel)

Kifa Clips

Two pairs of forceps, one of which should be dressing forceps, are required to remove Kifa clips.

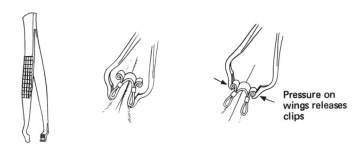

Pressure on wings releases clips

As one pair steadies the clip the wings of the clip are pressed together with the second pair of forceps.

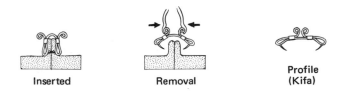

Inserted   Removal   Profile (Kifa)

The pointed ends of the clip then rise free of the skin and are removed.
N.B.

Nurse should always have a swab ready when removing sutures or clips so that they can be placed on it after removal and none are lost in the bed to cause discomfort to the patient.

When a patient has more than one wound, for example, a stitch line and a separate drainage wound, these should be dressed independently of each other.

Drains

Drains are used to drain fluid or air from the tissues, duct or cavity, for example, pus or serum may be drained from tissues, bile from the common bile duct or urine from the urinary tract and air from pleural cavity. What ever the reason, adequate instructions are given regarding their care and removal, and this guidance must be followed by the nurse. A note must be made in the patient's record of the presence of a drain. If and when it is shortened or removed this should also be noted in the records.

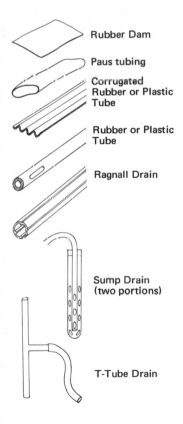

Rubber Dam

Paus tubing

Corrugated Rubber or Plastic Tube

Rubber or Plastic Tube

Ragnall Drain

Sump Drain (two portions)

T-Tube Drain

Wound drains are made of several types or styles of material. They can be made of fine sheet rubber or soft latex rubber tubing, corrugated sheet rubber or rubber tubing with or without holes in it. These drains would drain into dressings over the wound or into a colostomy type drainage bag.

Catheters and tubes may also be used and lathough some may drain into dressings, most are on closed drainage and may have suction applied, for example, after a mastectomy. If the drainage is from the pleural cavity a special type of drain called a water seal drain would be used.

Further details of the care of water seal drainage will be given in the section on "Thoracic Surgery". T-tube drainage is described in detail in the section on post operative care of a patient after choledochostomy. Drains are held in place by a suture or prevented from slipping back into the wound by the use of a sterile safety pin. They may be shortened before removal to prevent tissue damage and to encourage healing from the depth of the wound. When shortened they are drawn out from the wound for the required distance. If a suture is holding the tube or tubing, this is cut prior to shortening of the drain. A sterile safety pin is inserted into the tubing next to the skin using forceps and the excess tubing or corrugated rubber is then cut off using scissors. Great care must be taken to keep the skin surrounding a drainage tube or tubes clean and dry.

SPECIAL CARE

11

Intravenous Therapy or Transfusion

An intravenous infusion is the introduction of a fairly large amount of fluid into a patient's vein. A transfusion is the introduction or infusion of whole human blood or a derivative, such as plasma or cells, into the patient's vein. The fluid used in infusion is specially prepared and is a sterile solution so must not be contaminated in any way before the solution gets into the patient's blood stream. When blood is given it is carefully matched to the patient's own blood by doctor checking that the group is the same, that the Rhesus factor matches, and that to the best of his knowledge all other constituents of the blood match up.

Reasons for Infusion

The reasons for giving a patient an infusion are, first of all to replace lost fluids and salts. If the patient has had severe diarrhoea, has haemorrhaged, is having his stomach emptied by gastric suction or has been vomiting, he will lose a great deal of fluid and salts and may require infusion to replace them. The other main reason for giving an intravenous infusion is, as an alternative to the oral route of feeding. This may be used for the patient who has some disturbance of the alimentary tract or for the unconscious patient. A transfusion is given to replace blood or part of it, when for example the patient has haemorrhaged, is shocked, has lost fluid from burns or in the treatment of some anaemias.

The procedure of setting up an infusion or transfusion is the responsibility of the doctor who will be assisted by a nurse. Briefly the procedure is as follows.

Setting up an Infusion

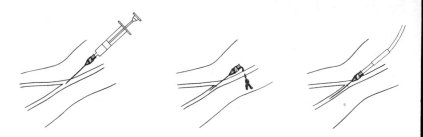

After the doctor has cleansed the patient's skin, a hollow needle or fine tube, which of course must be sterile, is introduced into the patient's vein and secured in position.

An infusion set attached to a bottle is used to transmit the fluid from the bottle to the patient. The tubing or giving set consists of clear tubing on the course of which is a drip chamber.

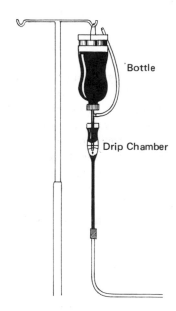

Bottle

Drip Chamber

The doctor decides the type and the amount of fluid which has to be given and the rate at which the fluid has to be delivered to the patient. This can be measured by counting the drops per minute in the drip chamber. Occasionally doctor has to expose a vein in order to set up an infusion (cut down).

The equipment for infusion would be the same as is required for an aseptic dressing with the addition of a disposable giving set with needle or cannula. To cut down on or expose a vein a special pack containing suturing material, scalpel, scissors, fine dissecting and "Mosquito" artery forceps, aneurysm needle, and blunt hook would be required.

Fluids used in Infusions

Sodium chloride (salt), potassium or dextrose are commonly used solutions given singly or in combination, in sterile distilled water. These solutions are prepared in pharmaceutical departments. Specially prepared solutions containing protein or fat are sometimes given.

Care of Blood

Blood is an extremely precious commodity and in Great Britain is donated free. It is therefore most important that the greatest of care is given to this gift to the patient. Blood should never be used straight from a refrigerator as it tends to be cold, but should be allowed to sit at room temperature for a little while prior to administration. It should never, under any circumstances, be stored in a food fridge as there is a strong possibility that the temperature of the food fridge is quite unsuitable for the storage of blood. A bottle of blood should never be shaken at any time or any active effort made to heat the blood.

Care of the Patient

Before and while the infusion is being set up, the patient should be given an explanation of the procedure.

Many patients and relatives are very apprehensive when infusions or transfusions are in progress, so nurse must take time to reassure them.

The general care of a patient must continue while intravenous therapy is in progress. The patient should be supported in a comfortable position suitable for the infusion. If the infusion is running into the

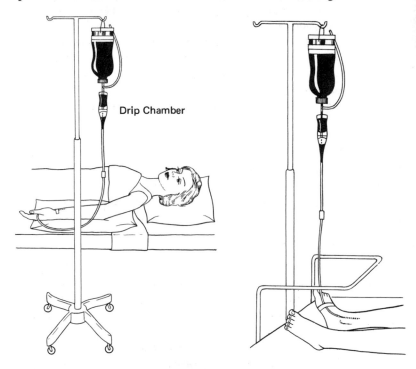

Drip Chamber

patient's arm it is supported on a covered pillow and if it is being delivered into a vein in the patient's leg a cage should support the bed clothes. The limb used should be kept warm to discourage spasm of the blood vessels which could stop the infusion. There should be no tension on the infusion set. The patient's locker should be within easy reach on the side not hindered by the infusion.

The patient should be dressed in a gown or night wear which will leave the arm or leg free and not necessitate the dangerous practice of removing garments and passing an intravenous bottle down sleeves or pyjama legs. Bed making may dislodge the needle if it is not carried out carefully. When the patient is being turned nurse should support the arm or leg into which the infusion is introduced. If the infusion is introduced into the patient's arm he may require assistance to keep his mouth clean and nurse must remember that some patients who are having intravenous fluids may also be allowed oral fluids and she should ascertain what is to happen. If oral fluids are allowed it is important that the nurse makes sure that they are given. The general hygiene of the patient should continue, and the patient will probably require assistance with, for example, brushing hair, general washing, getting on and off bed pans or help with using urinals. These little points, although they seem insignificant, should not be forgotten. A record must be kept of any fluid given and lost so that an accurate fluid balance chart is essential. Some authorities prefer blood or plasma to be charted separately from ordinary fluids and nurse should check therefore on the local practice in this connection.

Observation of the Infusion and the Site

The position of the stand should be such that it is not easily knocked over. The bottle or bag of infusion fluid must be securely hung from the stand so that it cannot be dislodged. Doctor will order the bottle of fluid so nurse should see that the next bottle which will be required is ready to put up when the one in use is almost empty. If a bandage or splints are used nurse should regularly check that they are in position. Any pain, redness, swelling, or leakage from the site of the needle should be reported to the nurse who is in charge of the ward. Any of these signs indicate that something has gone wrong with the infusion. If an infusion stops the nurse should check that the patient's limb is in the correct position and that the tubing is not kinked, but apart from these points she must not interfere with the infusion in any way but report the matter immediately to doctor who will deal with the problem.

Abnormal Reactions

Occasionally patients react adversely to the introduction of intravenous fluids into their veins. This is rather uncommon and if any reaction did occur it is more likely to do so if the patient was being given a transfusion. The signs which the nurse should be very careful to observe are as follows.

1. Any rise in the patient's temperature.

2. Any headache which the patient did not have prior to administration of the transfusion.

3. If the patient becomes shivery or complains of chest pain.

4. If he becomes more restless than he had been.

5. If he has difficulty in breathing or is coughing more than he was prior to the infusion.

All these observations should be made and if changes do occur these should be reported to the person in charge of the ward or to doctor, who will take the relevant steps to overcome the reaction. Occasionally a patient has a violent reaction to a transfusion, possibly due to the administration of the wrong blood, and in a situation like this the infusion should be stopped immediately.

Changing of the Bottle

A senior nurse is responsible for changing an intravenous infusion bottle, but she may require the assistance of a junior nurse to check several details in connection with this. The correct bottle, and the rate of flow, will be ordered by the doctor. It is important to observe the bottle at all times and the junior should report to the senior nurse when the level of fluid in the bottle is becoming low.

If it is an ordinary infusion bottle, which is being changed, the nurse will require to check that the correct bottle is being put up in place of the one which is almost empty and that the rate of flow is that ordered by doctor.

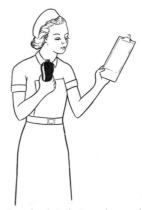

If on the other hand it is a transfusion bottle which is being changed it is equally important that care is taken in the changing of it but there are more stringent precautions to be followed. On each bottle or package of

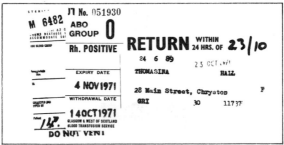

blood will be noted the patient's name, address and age, blood group and rhesus factor, and the expiry date of the blood. It is vital that two people, one a registered nurse or doctor, should check these details against the identity of the patient in bed and a check can be made on this by reference to the patient's identity bracelet and also to the details given on his case sheet. Blood should never be used after the expiry date. It must be returned to the blood transfusion department. Only when these have all been thoroughly checked should the bottle be changed, and again this is the responsibility of the senior nurse. If it is a blood package or bottle which is being changed a few millilitres of the blood should be left in the container for return to the blood transfusion department.

12
Oxygen Therapy

The aim in giving any patient oxygen is to increase the amount of oxygen in the air breathed which will then travel in solution in the blood to the blood cells. In a surgical ward a patient may require oxygen because he is very shocked, has lost a large amount of blood, or as a result of a head injury or on return from theatre.

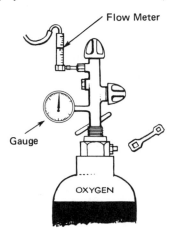

Oxygen is supplied in cylinders which are black in colour and have white shoulders as illustrated. A valve to regulate the escape of oxygen is situated at the upper end and is opened by using a key. Oxygen rushes out when the key is turned so it is important that the attachments necessary for delivering oxygen to the patient are attached and checked before oxygen is administered. A flow-meter allows control of the rate of oxygen flow to the patient. Oxygen can also be supplied via pipes in the ward and nurse must check that she attaches the tubing to the correct outlet. Oxygen has a drying effect on mucous membranes and is therefore humidified before administration, and this can be done by bubbling the oxygen through water.

Oxygen, in itself, is not inflammable but it supports combustion therefore precautions must be taken. No naked flames, cigarettes, or mechanical toys which could spark, should be used anywhere near oxygen and notices should be displayed to this effect. Patients on either side of the patient receiving the oxygen and any visitors should be advised of the danger. Grease or oil should never be used to lubricate joints or fittings on the oxygen equipment as this can cause an explosion. It is important that the oxygen gauge is observed as this will indicate to the nurse how much oxygen is left in the cylinder and she must make sure that this never becomes empty as the oxygen supply is then cut off to the patient and if the patient has a mask in position the patient could quite easily smother. A new cylinder should always be on hand and the seal should be checked to make sure that it is intact. Chalking the word "empty" on used cylinders cuts down any confusion during their use. The dosage of oxygen is decided and ordered by doctor at so many litres per minute and it is the nurse's duty to see that the ordered amount is registering on the flowmeter.

Choice of Method of Administration

The choice of method depends on several factors
1. The patient's condition
2. The concentration of oxygen required
3. The facilities available
4. The patient's ability to co-operate
5. The doctor's personal preference

But no matter the choice made, an adequate oxygen supply must be maintained.

There are three main groups of methods whereby oxygen may be administered.

1. Nasal Catheters and Oxygen Spectacles

Firstly it may be supplied via tubes inserted into the nostrils, for example, nasal catheter or oxygen spectacles. After explaining to the patient, his nose should be cleaned, the equipment tested by allowing oxygen to flow through it, the catheter should be lubricated with a water based lubricant and then passed up the nostril for approximately 5 centimetres. The catheter should be secured to the face with adhesive or if spectacles are being used these should be placed in position. The

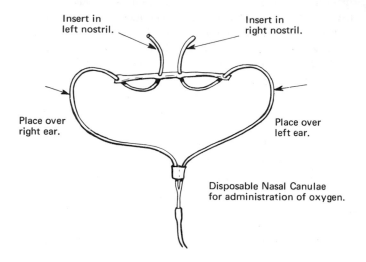

Insert in left nostril.

Insert in right nostril.

Place over right ear.

Place over left ear.

Disposable Nasal Canulae for administration of oxygen.

tubes or catheters should be changed every 48 to 72 hours or if they become blocked with discharge. The oxygen tubing used to connect to the supply should be supported with, for example, a pin attached to the bed clothes to give the patient some freedom of movement without a pull on the tubing. The tubing used should be of the anti static rubber variety which is normally black with a yellow line along the side. After use, the catheter or the tubing from the spectacles must be washed and sterilised if these are not disposable.

2. Masks

The next group which can be used are masks. These should cover the nose and the mouth or merely the nose, and are fixed in position by straps which secure the mask to the head. No matter what type is used, it should fit comfortably on the patient's face, otherwise he will not tolerate it and particularly with a confused patient, will try to remove it. A mask has the disadvantage that the patient is not able to speak, neither can he eat or drink, when it is in position, if it is of the type covering the nose and mouth. The advantage is that, with some masks, it is possible to be really sure that the correct percentage of oxygen is received by the patient.

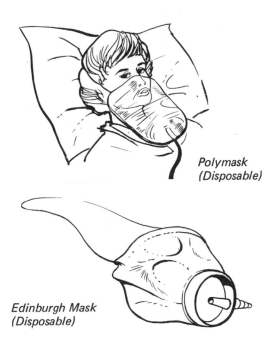

*Polymask
(Disposable)*

*Edinburgh Mask
(Disposable)*

3. Oxygen-filled Areas

A third method of administering oxygen is to have an area filled with oxygen. For example, this can be done by using an oxygen tent which consists of a clear canopy suspended over the bed and is tucked into the bed clothes. An attached unit cools the oxygen, humidifies it to the required extent and propels the oxygen into the tent by means of an electric motor. Closable openings are available to allow the nurse to insert her arms into the canopy to give the patient nursing care. The oxygen content can be kept at a constant level. The oxygen is turned on prior to use and then regulated to a steady flow. Most of the modern oxygen tents have a temperature control and the temperature is kept at around 18·3 degrees centigrade. An alternative method is by using an incubator where the same principles are applied, and is used for the small child.

The incubators come in several different styles and types but incorporate much the same features as have been mentioned for the oxygen tent. They also incorporate an alarm system whereby, if any unit of supply in the incubator should fail, an alarm bell rings and a light goes on.

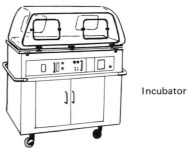

Incubator

Oxygen is occasionally given under pressure in association with some surgical care required by a patient. This would be done in a special chamber called a hyperbaric oxygen chamber and only specially trained personnel would be in charge and nurse in this area.

Care of the Patient

Patients receiving oxygen may be irritable, apprehensive or confused and unable to understand the explanation given. It may be necessary to repeat the instructions to him and much tact and patience is required when dealing with a patient who does not understand the necessity of oxygen administration.

Oxygen is required by each cell in the body for any activity it has to carry out so care should be taken to allow only permitted activity of the patient so that the cells do not exceed the supply of oxygen which the body is able to give to them.

The patient should be placed in a position which makes breathing easy for him and this often in an upright or semi-upright position. The ventilation of the ward or the room in which the patient is nursed must be adequate, but there should be no draughts.

Any item which the patient may require and is allowed to stretch for should be handy on his locker and it should be carefully placed at the side of his bed. Items such as a hanky or a glass of water should always be handy and the patient should have some means, such as a bell, to communicate with the nurse when he requires attention.

Restlessness is unnecessary activity which increases the use of oxygen in the body and can be caused by many factors of which discomfort is an important one.

Discomfort may arise from a badly made bed, uncomfortable position, full bladder, dry mouth, soiled clothing or feeling unwashed. Nurse must remedy this by making the bed, placing the patient in a comfortable position, give facilities for emptying the bladder, cleaning the mouth, changing clothing and attending to general hygiene.

Strain or stress also increases the body's demand for oxygen. An adequate diet or laxative may relieve the patient of the stress of constipation while medical, nursing and ancillary staff can help relieve anxiety regarding the patient's illness or home circumstances. A surfeit of visitors can tire the patient, so short visiting spells should be enforced. Loud noises are stress provoking so nurses must work quietly and efficiently. Televisions and radios should be quietened or removed.

Observation of the Patient

While the patient is receiving oxygen he requires to be carefully observed. In the first half-hour of oxygen administration particular observation of the patient should be carried out. This observation should be of the rate and depth of breathing, the temperature and colour of the skin and the quality of the pulse.

Nurse should also report any difficulty in breathing which the patient did not have prior to oxygen administration, if the patient complains of a pain behind the sternum (breast bone) or if the patient looks as if he is becoming more drowsy than he was previously.

If the patient begins to look a little blue (cyanosed), nurse should check that there is no kink in the tubing, that the oxygen supply has not run out, and that the mask is not disconnected from the supply. If any of these eventualities occur the patient using a mask or in a tent could suffocate.

Any abnormal signs must be reported immediately.

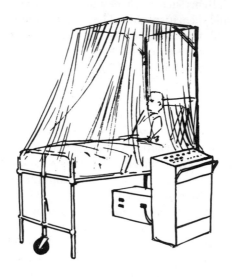

13
Suction

Suction apparatus may be required to clear secretions from a patient's nose or mouth, to aspirate gastric secretions or to prevent the collection of fluid in a wound.

In a ward, low suction may be available using a Roberts Pump or there may be machines capable of more powerful suction such as the Matburn Machine or pipe-line suction.

Machines should be maintained by a technician or electrician and any faults in them or in the plug and cable in the electric pumps should be reported so that skilled repair can be carried out. Machines must be tested before use and must not be used if faulty as the nurse or patient is then exposed to danger.

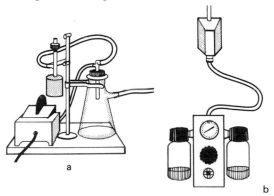

a) *Portable Robert's suction pump.*
b) *Fixed wall suction.*

Pressure tubing should be used to maintain satisfactory suction. Ordinary tubing is liable to kink. The connection used to attach the suction tubing to the catheter or tube at the patient's end should be well fitting and of the clear unbreakable variety. The bottle into which the aspirate is received should be firmly sealed so that a vacuum is maintained.

As the secretions aspirated may be infected the jar and tubing should be thoroughly washed and rinsed after use prior to sterilisation either by autoclaving or by chemicals.

Doctor will order the level of suction required and nurse must observe the machine to see that the level is maintained. Low suction at 2 − 5 centimetres of mercury (Hg.) would probable be required for wound or gastric suction while aspiration of secretions from nose and mouth would probably require a higher level.

The nurse must always observe and note the amount, character, colour, and quantity of the fluid aspirated. Nurse should also make sure that the aspirate is not required for inspection by doctor or a senior nurse before it is discarded.

Nasal and Oral Suction

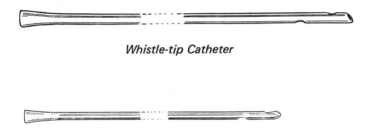

Whistle-tip Catheter

Jacques Catheter

To aspirate the nose and mouth a sterile Jacques or whistle-tipped catheter may be used. This may be rinsed by sucking a measured amount of fresh water through it between aspirations. This amount would be deducted from the total aspirate before entering the quantity on the fluid balance chart.

Gastric Suction

When the patient's stomach is being emptied the suction tubing is attached to the naso-gastric tube using a clear non-breakable connection. The gastric suction may be either continuous or intermittent. If it is continuous gastric suction which is being employed the suction machine should be switched off for five minutes in the hour to prevent the end of the tube becoming adherent to the stomach wall. Intermittent gastric suction will vary in the length of time it is employed, from five minutes in the hour to ten or fifteen minutes in the hour. To prevent

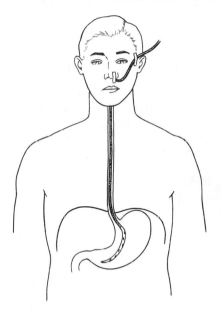

the tube dragging on the patient's nose it is strapped first of all to the patient's cheek and then the suction tubing is pinned onto the patient's pillow in such a way that it does not cause restriction of the patient's movement.

Wound Suction

A catheter or tube is fixed into the wound at operation and the suction apparatus is attached with a well fitting, non-breakable connection on return to the ward. Sometimes a container inside which

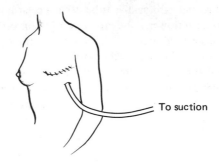

Wound suction via stab wound

is a vacuum, for example, a Redivac Drain, is attached to the wound catheter and in this way suction is applied. Wound suction should always be at a low level of suction and is mostly about two centimetres of mercury.

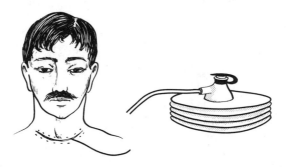

Wound suction — to disposable vacuum suction apparatus

14
Nutrition

Food is nutritive material and may come in solid or liquid form and as such is taken into the body. Food is necessary for life and although some people may live to eat it is equally true that one must eat to enable one to live!

Food is necessary for normal body function, to provide fuel for energy, to supply materials for growth and repair of the body tissues and to protect the body from disease.

The food which is eaten comes from animal and vegetable sources and the body is rather wonderfully constructed to prepare this food so that each individual cell of the body can make use of it. A person must receive and utilise this food from his diet and only if he can do this will he be well nourished. To be well nourished the diet must contain the following items:

1. protein so that the body can grow and repair itself and also to a certain extent provide a source of energy.

2. fat so that the individual has energy for doing his work and fat also supports and protects some of the organs of the body.

3. carbohydrate provides another source of energy and body fat

4. water which is necessary for all body functions

5. mineral salts, which are necessary for the regulation of the various body processes and are also helpful in the growth and repair of the body.

6. vitamins, which are essential for protection against disease and aid in regulation of body function.

If all these items are present in their proper proportions in the diet the patient or the person is said to be having a well balanced diet. If this is so his body should be well developed. He should be of average weight for his body size. His skin, hair and eyes should be healthy. His posture should be good. He should be mentally alert.

A Calorie is the unit which is used to measure the amount of energy which can be obtained from the different foodstuffs taken in in the diet. Fat would yield more than twice as much energy and heat from the same amount of food composed of either carbohydrate or protein. Foods are valued according to the amount of heat and energy they produce when used in the body.

Food is necessary from birth to death, but the needs of the individual will vary depending on his age and on the amount of activity which he is called upon to perform. A patient in bed may therefore require less calories than a manual labourer.

In disease the normal eating habits of a person may be changed either because his illness makes him disinclined for food, as part of his treatment or as part of his pre- or post-operative care. Although the variety or number of diets given in a surgical ward may be less than in a medical situation they are still important.

Diet Therapy

Diet therapy is a modification of a normal diet to meet the requirements of a sick individual.

There are several aims in giving diets to a patient and the following are a selection of the main ones —

1. To maintain good nutritional status
2. To increase or decrease weight
3. To allow a particular organ of the body to rest (e.g. restriction of fat in gall bladder disease)
4. To remedy a deficiency (e.g. rickets)
5. To eliminate harmful substances from the diet (e.g. condiments or roughage in some conditions of the gastro-intestinal tract)

The diet can be modified in several ways. The calorie value may be increased or decreased. The balance of the various nutrients, that is, the amounts of carbohydrate, fat and protein may be adjusted. If the patient is allergic to particular foods these would be omitted from the diet. The diet can also be modified in consistency, for example, a diet taken by an ordinary individual would include fluids and solids, for a sick individual a semi solid or a completely fluid diet might be necessary.

For any person who is receiving a diet it is important that it is presented to them in an attractive fashion. The food must be

arranged on spotlessly clean utensils in portions of suitable size.
It should not be lacking in colour. The person presenting the food
to the patient should be of a pleasant disposition and should make
sure that all the cutlery which the patient will require and any
condiments allowed are on the tray before she gives it to the patient.
Only one course should be served at a time and soiled dishes must
be removed prior to each serving. Each patient should be treated as
an individual and with a little care and consideration foods which the
patient dislikes, but are not necessarily harmful to him, may be
omitted from the diet so that he may really enjoy his meals. Hot
foods or fluids should be served hot, cold food or fluids should be
served cold not warm. Many patients will require to be fed and
it is essential that the person doing this sits in a comfortable position,
if possible, has the patient also in a comfortable position and
takes her time to feed the patient at the rate at which the patient
requires to be fed. Patience and kindliness are essential in feeding a
helpless patient.

Diets

An Ordinary Diet

This would be eaten by a patient needing no modification in his
diet. It will contain protein in food such as meat, fish, eggs, cheese,
carbohydrate from sugar or starches such as potatoes and flour. Fat
which takes longer to digest, comes from cream, butter, fish oils and
margarine. Water which is found in many foods as well as in its natural
form. Vitamins, minerals and roughage will also be required and will
be found in the following foods. Vitamins A, D, E, K, mainly in fatty
foods such as eggs, milk and fish liver oils, vitamin B in yeast, liver,
eggs and some vegetables, vitamin C in green vegetables and fresh
fruit such as blackcurrants, oranges and lemons. Roughage is the part
of food which the body is unable to digest and is found in fruit,
vegetables and whole meal foods. It provides bulk to the diet and thus
helps to satisfy the appetite and maintain normal bowel function.

Light Diet

This diet is one which is easily digested by the patient and
would be given for a few days prior to operation. It is also given in the

post-operative period as a stage in the patient's return to his normal diet.

Low Residue Diet

This provides the patient with the desired nourishment but includes very little roughage and excludes foods with a laxative action such as prunes. It would be given on the days prior to operation on the bowel or before barium examination. It is also given to patients who have inflammatory disease of the bowel or have diarrhoea. Post-operatively after bowel operation it would be used as a stage in the return to normal diet or, after a haemorrhoidectomy, it would help to confine the bowel.

Fluid Diets

Patients who have difficulty in swallowing may require a fluid diet. This must be carefully prepared to make sure that the patient has a balanced diet. It is also important that variety is introduced, as a succession of milky drinks of the same flavour can be very boring and nauseating to the patient. "Complan", "Carnation" breakfast food, "Marmite", "Bovril", "Horlicks", "Ovaltine", coffee, chocolate, switched egg, and fruit juices should be alternated. It cannot be stressed enough that this must be a carefully planned diet or the patient may not receive sufficient nourishment. The use of clear soups or liquidised foods can add variety and provide additional nourishment. A patient who is having a fluid diet in hospital must always have a record of intake and output kept on a fluid balance chart. Post operatively when some patients are allowed only water orally, nourishment would be supplied by the alternative route of intravenous infusion.

Reduction Diets

Prior to surgery it may be necessary to have a patient on a diet in order to reduce his weight. Sweet foods are not given but protein foods and a limited amount of fats are supplied. When a patient is on a reduction diet he should be weighed at regular intervals.

Low Fat Diet

A patient who has disease of the liver or gall bladder may have a low fat diet given to him as part of his treatment, pre- or post-operatively. The bile produced by the liver and stored in the gall bladder is necessary for digestion and absorption of fat. If there is any disturbance to the flow of this bile, the body cannot cope adequately with the fat, therefore the amount of it in the diet requires to be reduced.

Diabetic Diet

Each Diabetic patient has a diet specially tailored to his needs. The diet would have reduced amounts of carbohydrate compared to an ordinary diet. The consistency of the diet would be varied, depending on the patient's needs after operation.

General Instructions

It is important if a patient is on a diet that he knows he is on one, he is given the reason for his diet and his relatives are also advised so that they do not bring undesirable food, sweets, fluids or titbits into the hospital. The importance of adhering to the diet should be stressed to the patient. It is particularly important when the patient is on a reducing diet as the patient needs much will power and encouragement to stick to the diet.

Serving Food

Whatever the diet, it is essential that it be served in an attractive and appetizing way. Most surgical patients, both before and after operation, have poor appetites and require to be tempted to start eating. Small, easily managed portions served in an attractive manner are the best way to stimulate the gastric juices.

Artificial Methods of Feeding

The patient is sometimes unable to eat or swallow a normal or modified diet and may require to be fed by tube. The tube may be passed via the nose and oesophagus into the stomach. Sometimes a special tube is introduced through the abdominal wall into the stomach to allow feeding of the patient. This requires an operation called a gastrostomy. Fluid is occasionally given into the rectum but very little absorption takes place from here so solutions used are restricted to glucose, water and salt. Other possible routes are subcutaneous infusion when fluid is introduced into the tissues or intravenous infusion when it is delivered into a vein.

The fluids given via naso-gastric tube or gastrostomy tube would be similar to those mentioned for the fluid diet. Prior to administering the fluid by naso-gastric tube a syringe would be attached to the end of it and a little of the stomach secretion withdrawn. As the stomach contents are normally acid this fluid should turn blue litmus paper to red. If this is not so the nurse must report the matter and should refrain from giving the feed until she has further instructions. The fluid is given by funnel attached to a tube at a temperature of 38 degrees centigrade. Approximately 50 millilitres of water is often introduced into the tube before and after the feed to keep the tube clear.

The patient lies on his left side or in a sitting up position while the feed is being given. On completion a clean spiggot is inserted in the end of the tube.

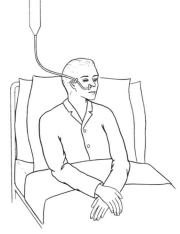

Feeding via Gastrostomy Tube

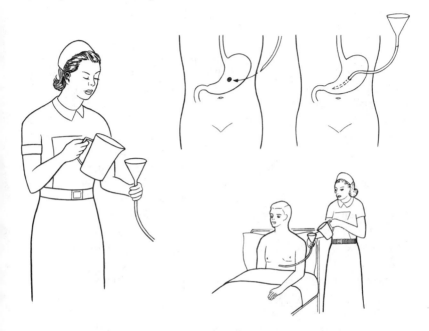

If the feed is given to the patient via a gastrostomy tube the area of skin surrounding it should be carefully cleansed so that any acid gastric juice can be cleared away and thus prevent digestion of the skin of the abdominal wall.

A patient who is being fed artificially must always have a record kept of the fluid which is given and a fluid balance chart is kept. If a naso-gastric tube is being used to feed the patient the nasal passages must be kept clean to prevent crusting around the tube and subsequent discomfort to the patient. The patient's mouth will require very careful cleaning as he is not chewing in the normal fashion. After feeding, the funnel, tubing and connection are washed and dried thoroughly ready for the next feed. When the patient no longer requires feeding in this manner this equipment, if not disposable, would be sterilised before use by another patient.

15
The Unconscious Patient

A patient who is aware of what is happening around him is said to be conscious. When he is not fully aware of his surroundings, but is not merely asleep, he is said to be unconscious. Consciousness is described in degrees or depth and sometimes terms such as semiconscious or stupor are used in an attempt to state the level of consciousness. A small child paddling in a foot of water may say that the pond is deep, but the same depth will be shallow to his father, so with terms such as "semi-conscious" it may mean different things to different people. It is therefore safer to describe the patient's level of awareness by describing his reaction to attempts to rouse him. In this way a more accurate record is kept and improvement or otherwise can be recognised. Since one patient may be cared for by several different nurses in the course of 24 hours clearly understandable observations are important.

There are many causes of unconsciousness, such as diabetes mellitus, epilepsy, cerebrovascular accidents or a simple faint. In a surgical ward, however, the common causes are head injuries of all kinds, unconscious-ness following anaesthesia or failed resuscitation. The care of an unconscious patient must include the treatment and investigation of its cause. This will be dealt with in the section under Head Injury, but the general basic care of an unconscious patient varies little with its cause, only the amount of care required will vary.

An ordinary individual is able to breath feed, move, keep himself clean, change his clothes, control bodily excretions, protect himself from injury, communicate with others, identify himself appreciate his surroundings and keep himself healthy. The ability of a patient who is not fully conscious to do these things is impaired. The ward staff must therefore be responsible for meeting his needs. The amount of basic care he will require will depend on how long unconsciousness lasts. Any patient who is unconscious needs someone to make sure that his airway is kept clear, but the patient who merely faints will not require attention to personal hygiene as will the patient whose head injury may have kept him unconscious for weeks.

An unconscious patient must never be left unattended at any time and must have an identity bracelet or some other means of identification attached on admission so that mistakes regarding his identity in administration of drugs or treatments may be avoided.

Airway

To make sure that the patient gets sufficient oxygen and gets rid of carbon dioxide there must be a clear route from his nose and mouth right to his lungs.

The patient may be unable to cough and swallow so special care must be taken. The things which might block his airway are

1. Secretions from nose or mouth
2. The patient's tongue falling backwards
3. Artificial dentures becoming dislodged
4. Vomitus being inhaled
5. Secretions gathering in the lung
6. Careless tube feeding, when fluid may be introduced into the lungs instead of the stomach
7. Bed clothes or pillows, if carelessly placed, can smother the patient.

To prevent the occurence of these situations the following measures should be taken. The patient should be positioned in the semi-prone or lateral position with his head at a lower level than his feet and his tongue lying forward. Physiotherapy and careful turning from side to side will help to prevent the occurrence of hypostatic pneumonia. Secretions or vomitus draining via nose and mouth can be sucked out using a suction catheter. Care during tube feeding and bedmaking will prevent an inhalation pneumonia or smothering of the patient. Dentures should be removed to avoid blockage to the air passages. The patient should be nursed at all times on a firm mattress as a sagging mattress predisposes to the collection of secretions in the lungs and leads to chest complications.

After an anaesthetic an artificial airway may be inserted to keep the airway clear and it also prevents the patient's tongue from falling backwards. If the patient is unconscious for more than two or three days he may have an artifical opening made in his trachea and a tube introduced. This is called a tracheostomy. A patient who has a tracheostomy requires very special care as he can easily develop a chest infection or block his tube.

The Skin

One of the biggest challenges in the care of an unconscious patient is to keep a healthy skin. To do this the patient must be kept spotlessly clean and dry at all times. Pressure sores or bed sores are one of the biggest problems which have to be faced in the care of the skin of an unconscious patient.

There are four main factors which cause pressure sores:-

1. Pressure
2. Friction
3. Moisture
4. Inadequate nutrition

Pressure

Whether in nursing school or at home, if a person sits listening to a lecture or watching television he changes his position regularly, as otherwise he becomes very uncomfortable and sore. An unconscious patient is not aware of this happening and he could stay in any particular position and develop sores. The circulation to the parts of the body on which there is pressure is cut off and the tissues are unable to receive adequate oxygen and nourishment from the blood and are therefore damaged or die.

The patient will be nursed in various positions. These would probably be, left semi-prone, prone, right semi-prone and lateral positions in turn. The nurses must be aware of the fact that pressure sores can be caused by the patient's own weight, not only on the sacrum and heels but also on knees, toes, ankles, feet, elbows, shoulders, head, hips and over the spine if he lies in one position for too long a period of time. Pressure may also come from tight bed clothes, sand bags and bed cages. Beds must therefore have a wrinkle free sheet and perhaps also a draw sheet under the patient. The upper bed clothes should be supported by a bed cage carefully positioned so that it does not cause pressure on the patient's legs. Sand bags, if used, should be carefully positioned to make sure there is no pressure on the patient. A mattress made of large air cells which alternately inflate and deflate helps to relieve pressure on the skin. A timetable made of positions in which the patient should lie is helpful as it gives a guide and provides a record of when the patient should be turned and in what position he should lie at any particular time.

CYCLE FOR TURNING

Position	Position of Feet	Time	Mon	Tue	Wed	Thur	Fri	Sat	Sun
LEFT LATERAL		4 AM							
		NOON							
		20.00 HRS							
DORSAL		6 AM							
		14.00 HRS							
		22.00 HRS							
RIGHT LATERAL		8 AM							
		16.00 HRS							
		24.00 HRS							
PRONE		10 AM							
		18.00 HRS							
		2 AM							

Friction

This means the rubbing together of two structures. Friction may be caused by bad lifting techniques. If instead of two or more nurses lifting the patient clear of the bed he is pulled or dragged from one position to another his skin is rubbed against the bed clothes and can be damaged. Two skin surfaces rubbing together, for example, the inner aspects of the knees, may also damage the skin. If a nurse is careless in the administration of bed pans and pushes them under the patient rather than lifting the patient clear and sitting him on the bed pan, the skin can be broken.

Moisture

The body rids itself of some of its waste products through the skin so great care should be taken to make sure that two damp skin surfaces are not constantly lying together. The groins, fold of the buttocks and under pendulous breasts are sites where this may occur. These areas should be carefully washed and dried.

The skin may become soiled by urinary or faecal incontinence, after administration of an enema or become damp due to the use of a wet bedpan. The skin should always be washed and dried if soiling occurs and if the patient is incontinent the use of a barrier cream is often recommended after cleansing.

Vaginal discharge not only causes moisture but also irritation and for this doctor would order special treatment.

The patient should always have any soiled personal or bed linen changed when required and never at any time be left in damp or soiled clothing.

Inadequate Nutrition

The patient may be malnourished on admission and his skin may be in an unhealthy state. It is therefore necessary that while in hospital patients are adequately nourished. Any deficiencies in the diet should be corrected during the stay in hospital.

Patients are sometimes inadequately nourished in hospital because of carelessness on the part of nursing staff. This is particularly so when a patient is being nourished by fluid feeds and nurses may forget to give the patient the fluids he requires or think that fluid in the form of water is sufficient. It is therefore necessary that an unconscious patient, since he is not receiving an ordinary diet, is carefully observed as to the amount and the character of any fluid given and that in each day he has a well balanced diet.

Other Factors

Other factors known to predispose to the formation of "pressure sores" are patients who have injury or disease of nerves or blood vessels and if this is so the patient is more likely to develop pressure sores than a patient with other diseases. The skin may also be damaged by trauma. Nurses who wear wrist watches and stoned rings while attending to patients are liable to graze or cut the patient's skin, these should therefore never be worn. Hot water bottles are a menace as the patient who is unconscious is unaware of the heat and could easily become burned so they should never be used in the nursing of unconscious patients. Nurses' and patient's nails can tear the skin so these should be kept clean and short at all times.

A pressure sore can develop in a very short space of time, (e.g. a patient who has a fractured spine if pressure is not relieved by change of position within the first two hours after injury a sore is a likely outcome). A pressure sore appears as red, tender, painful area and if the pressure on the part is not relieved, the skin will break down. This stage is followed by a stage when the skin tissues become more congested and appear rather like a bruise or have a mottled appearance and the patient at this stage feels no pain. If the situation is allowed to continue the skin will break. It is very difficult to keep a "bed sore" free from contamination and many become infected. If this is so and a small sore becomes a massive sore the patient may become so ill that he may die from the toxins from this sore rather than from his original illness. If the situation is not as bad as this the patient will certainly have to prolong his stay in hospital and this may have financial implications for his family and can affect his home circumstances.

Treatment

There are a variety of ways in which bed sores are treated, but the important thing is that each treatment must fit the need of the individual patient. No matter what treatment is suggested for the patient pressure on the particular broken area must be relieved and the patient must have a good, well balanced diet. The pressure sore must be dressed with aseptic precautions, no matter the site of the sore. Sometimes doctor decides that local treatment using powders, ointments or solutions is insufficient and a skin graft may be applied for some patients. This would receive the same care as any skin graft.

General Hygiene

The unconscious patient, like any person, requires washing. The patient is unable to do this for himself and therefore this is another task which the nurse must perform for him. The patient must be bathed regularly and the frequency of this well depend on how much soiling there is of the patient, and of course on the condition of his skin.

The genital area needs special attention when bathing the patient as it is normally moist and if neglected can become very smelly and the skin can become excoriated. It is important though, that an excess of soap is not used as this, in the female, can damage the delicate mucous membrane of the vulva and vagina.

The patient's hair must be kept tidy. If he or she is unconscious for a long period of time, and depending on the cause of the unconsciousness it may be possible to wash the patient's hair or to clean it by using a dry shampoo. After it has been cleaned it should be neatly arranged in, if possible, the patient's usual style.

Sometimes the unconscious patient is also paralysed in some or many parts of his body. If for example his eye will not close on its own the cornea must be protected. The eyelids may be taped using a tiny piece of adhesive or micropore tape. This should be removed regularly during the day and night to allow observation of the eye. Doctor may order the installation of eye drops, irrigation or application of ointment.

Ears should be kept clean by normal washing and only in situations where there is a discharge would doctor order mopping or cleansing of the ear to be carried out. Special instructions would be given if there was discharge from the ear of a patient who had a head injury, but normally this would not be mopped out.

If a person is conscious he can generally wipe his own nose, but the unconscious patient must have this attended to for him. The nurse must clean it perhaps using "Q-Tips" or a wooden probe with its end covered in cotton wool to cleanse the nostrils gently.

Many unconscious patients breathe through their mouth therefore the mouth requires special care. If the patient has artificial dentures these would be removed on admission, cleaned, labelled, and stored in a safe place. If the patient still has his own teeth, these would be cleaned using a tooth brush and the patient's mouth swabbed out regularly to keep it moist and free from infection. Cleansing solutions should be used with care as excess fluid could be inhaled into the patient's lungs. The patient's head should be turned to the side while his mouth is being cleaned and if a suction catheter is available the danger of inhaled solution is cut down.

108

A solution of sodium bicarbonate is helpful in breaking down mucus and cleaning debris from the mouth, Glycerine of Thymol is useful as an antiseptic agent, Glycerine and lemon encourage the flow of saliva. To prevent cracking of the lips vaseline can be smeared thinly over them. When the patient's mouth is being cleaned, nurse should always use a torch and make sure that she inspects the mouth adequately to see that no ulceration or infection has developed since the last treatment.

Positioning and Moving the Patient

Lifting and turning of the patient is a necessary part of an unconscious patient's care. It helps prevent secretions gathering in the lungs, the formation of pressure sores, venous thrombosis, stagnation of urine in the bladder, ureter or kidneys, which of course would predispose to infection.

When lifting and turning a patient his limbs should be put through their

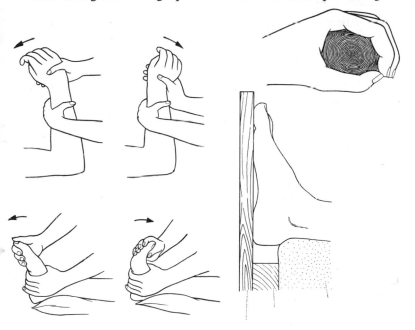

full range of movements to prevent wastage of muscles, contractures or stiff joints developing. Even if an unconscious patient is paralysed, his limbs must be positioned in such a way that they will be in a useful position on recovery. The joints should be placed in a position half way between flexion and extension, the foot supported at an angle of 90 degrees to the leg to avoid foot drop and the wrist supported. The physiotherapist can, in many hospitals, only give a limited amount of physiotherapy to each patient so the nurse must move the limbs through a range of passive exercises at every available opportunity. During the actual turning of the patient it is important that his spine is kept straight and if a turning sheet is used this may help to prevent wrong positioning and save strain both on the nurses and on the patient's muscles and frame. When positioning and moving the patient the condition of skin should be observed.

Nutrition

The patient may be fed by the intragastric or intravenous route. With the former, doctor would pass a naso-gastric tube into the stomach and small feeds of about 100 to 200 millilitres of solution would be administered every two to three hours. To keep the naso-gastric tube clear, 50 millilitres of water is often inserted before and after each feed. The tube would be changed regularly. A careful plan is made out for the patient's feeding regime and a balanced diet is given in fluid form and a record kept of the amounts and substances given. The nurse must always check the position of the tube prior to each feed and if she is in any doubt she must get the doctor to check. If the patient is being fed by the intravenous route, doctor orders all bottles of fluid or solution and indicates how long each should run and when each should be commenced.

Elimination

The waste of the body is excreted via the air leaving the lungs, the sweat from the skin, urine from the kidneys, and faeces from the bowel.

The skin can be washed to get rid of this waste, but from the kidneys, it is important that a note is made of the output of urine so that there is some indication whether or not the kidneys are functioning or perhaps if the urine is being retained in the bladder. Retention of urine in the bladder could be noted by the nurse observing distention of the abdomen. A catheter may be passed on the patient who is unconscious for a long time, but this is a decision which is not made lightly. If a catheter is not passed and the patient is incontinent of urine special care of the skin is necessary. With the male patient it may be possible to fit a special urinal to the penis and thus prevent excoriation of the skin and possible infection because of the introduction of a catheter. If a catheter is used the bladder may be drained on continuous drainage and it is the nurse's responsibility to see

1 That the tubing is not kinked at any time
2 That there is a free flow of urine from the bladder to the drainage bag.
3 That the drainage bag is replaced regularly with sterile precautions.
4. That it is always kept at a lower level than the bladder so that the urine drains into it and not from the bag to the bladder.

The bowel may be regulated by giving the patient a balanced diet by intragastric tube. Substances such as prune juice or a fluid aperient may be given at regular intervals so that the patient's bowel moves regularly. Suppositories or enemata are sometimes required to stimulate bowel function. The patient should be observed very carefully to make sure that he does not become constipated.

Observations

On admission and at all stages of the patient's unconsciousness he requires careful observation. These observations must be accurate, regular, detailed and are recorded on charts and in written reports.

One of the most important of the observations is the noting of the patient's level of consciousness and any change in level from the previous record should be noted and reported to sister or doctor. As the level of consciousness will vary from time to time and as it is often difficult to decide whether or not the patient is able to hear, it is therefore important that nurses and relatives do not converse or discuss the patient in his presence. This could have an adverse psychological effect on the patient. Nevertheless it may be helpful if the nurse speaks to the patient while caring for him.

The level of consciousness is assessed on the patient's response to his environment and various stimuli often described in four broad groups.

1. The patient who is fully conscious will respond to his surroundings and someone speaking to him
2. The patient will respond to simple commands but will not be fully conscious
3. The patient will respond to painful stimuli like the pricking of the patient with a pin
4. There is no obvious response at all even to painful stimuli

It is safer to describe the levels of consciousness rather than using numbers such as number one, two three and four or terms such as semi-conscious as there is a wide variation in the interpretation of these symbols and terms.

One of the observations which is helpful to doctor is the reaction obtained by shining a light from a pencil torch into each eye in turn and noting whether or not the patient's pupil constricts as the light is shone into it. Observations of the size of the pupil, whether or not it is dilated or constricted, if each pupil is the same size as the other or if there is any irregularity in the outline of the pupil may help doctor in his diagnosis and give him some indication of the patient's prognosis.

The temperature, pulse and respiratory rate recordings will be made at regular intervals as may the blood pressure estimation. These will give a guide to the general condition of the patient.

The temperature will be recorded rectally to ensure an accurate recording. While the patient is unconscious he is unable to control his temperature by the amount of clothing which he wears. This therefore must be done for him by the nurse and she should judge by the patient's temperature just how much clothing and bed clothing he requires. Naturally if the patient's temperature is exceptionally high he will require little or no covering. This would help to reduce the temperature.

If the temperature is raised well above normal levels the patient may require sponging with tepid water in an attempt to reduce the body temperature.

An accurate record must be kept of the fluid intake and output from this patient. This again will give doctor some indication of the amount of function that there is in the patient's kidneys and may also allow early recognition of any upset in kidney function. Other observations which should be made by the nurse during her care of the patient would include noting if there was any paralysis of any part of the body or if any paralysis previously present had disappeared, if there was any weakness of any of the voluntary muscle movements or if the patient suffered from tremors or convulsions. All these should be noted carefully and reported in written form so that any change in the amount of paralysis or the number of convulsions can be noted by doctor.

During any stage of the patient's illness it is important that treatment and any nursing care given to the patient is carried out in the accepted fashion of the hospital so that the patient comes to no harm during the treatments. During unconsciousness when the patient may suffer from convulsions, it is important that he does not injure himself. Nurse should therefore observe the patient very carefully to make sure that there are no objects that would harm him. An unconscious patient should have sides on the bed which would prevent him from falling out of it, but it is important that these sides should not be solid sides so that the nurse can observe the patient easily. If an unconscious patient becomes restless the nurse should check for any obvious cause such as a full bladder or awkward positioning of the patient. The patient may settle when these are corrected.

Continuing Care

After the initial stages of his illness, when very close observations must be made on the patient and intensive nursing care given, the patient may, depending on the length of his unconsciousness, require less frequent recordings but will still require a very high standard of regular nursing care.

When the patient begins to recover, his level of consciousness will vary and may do so quite considerably. For the patient who has been unconscious for a long period of time it is disturbing to realise that a period of time has passed during which he was unaware of the events taking place around him. The nursing staff must also realise that the level of consciousness will vary and because a patient becomes conscious does not mean that he can be left unattended. The conscious level can change quickly.

It is important that the patient is reorientated to his surroundings and to the staff. If the cause of the patient's unconsciousness was a head injury he may have been quite unaware of the fact of his admission to hospital and although this may be obvious to him on his return to consciousness an explanation is necessary. Exactly how much detail the patient would be given would depend on how much the doctor thought was advisable and necessary to his care. The patient, obviously, will need much encouragement and moral support from the nurse so that he will feel secure in hospital and will eventually be able to reorientate himself to a normal way of living. The patient may or may not have large gaps in his memory apart from anything that he may have missed when he was unconscious. It is important that the patient should not force himself to try to remember any particular phase in his life unless doctor specifically orders.

Rehabilitation has of course started from admission in that, during the nursing care of this patient, the nurse has attempted to keep his body in as fit a condition as possible so that when he recovers consciousness and is again able to begin moving his limbs himself they are not complicated by contractures, stiff joints or wasted muscles.

As a result of the period of unconsciousness it may be necessary for the patient to take up a new type of occupation. If this is so, the medical social workers, who would be contacted at the beginning of the patient's illness, would by the time the patient recovered consciousness be reasonably well acquainted with the patient's circumstances and would be able to help him in this particular situation. The disablement resettlement officer may be contacted as he would eventually be able to send the patient to an assessment centre so that his capabilities could be ascertained and a decision made on the type of employment which was most suited to his needs. However, it may be possible for the patient to return to his original job and the time at which he returned to this would very much depend on what doctor advised.

During the time of the patient's unconsciousness, during the recovery period and subsequent to his recovery of consciousness, the patient's relatives have a very worrying time. During the period of unconsciousness they will naturally be distressed by the appearance of their relative and the fact that they are unable to communicate with him. It is essential that they are reassured and given as much information as possible regarding the seriousness of the patient's condition and when or whether a change in the level of consciousness is expected. Despite the fact that the patient is initially unconscious it is important that the relatives do visit regularly so that the ward staff have a direct link with them through visiting and if possible they should have a telephone number available so that contact can be made quickly if there is any change in the patient's condition.

When relatives are visiting the hospital it is important that nurses remember that, to a certain extent, they are responsible for their health. A nurse should not allow a patient's relative to become over distressed, tired or exhausted by sitting at a patient's bedside and should make sure that the relative has a meal at the same time as the ward patients. If the relative is to stay at the hospital the nurse must ensure that the provision for her comfort is adequate and doctor may in fact order a sedative for the patient's relative so that he can have a good night's rest. During the time when the patient is unconscious the hospital chaplain, (no matter what denomination) or their own minister of religion, can often be of great comfort and help to the patient's relatives. Facilities should always be given to speak in privacy to the relatives.

It is important that the relatives realise that the level of consciousness of the patient will vary, particularly during the phase when he is returning to full consciousness. The reason for this is that the patient's relatives may become distressed at a regression to unconsciousness, and also from the patient's point of view the relatives may say something in his presence which he may very well be able to hear but to which he is unable to respond.

The surroundings in which the patient is nursed are important. Even although the patient is not aware of them, as far as is known, the effect on the staff of bright, tidy, clean surroundings makes them more cheerful and more optimistic and a like situation also applies to the patient's relatives. It also gives relatives a feeling that the staff really care for the patient and for them.

TERMINOLOGY

16
Understanding the Surgical Terms

At first sight many of the words used in surgery to describe conditions and operations are daunting. They are quite simple however if one breaks them into sections. The ending tells you what has been done or what the condition is, while the main part of the word tells you the organ or tissue involved. The following list gives the words and endings from which most common conditions and operations are derived.

Endings

— ITIS	Inflammation of
— OSIS	A condition of
— OTOMY	An opening into
— ECTOMY	Excision of
— OSTOMY	The formation of a new opening in (often to the skin surface)
— PLASTY	A reformation of
— GRAM	An x-ray picture of
— OMA	A tumour of

Main Stems

Trache	— Trachea	Hyster	— uterus
Bronch	— bronchus	Salping	— fallopian tubes
Pneumon	— lung	Hepat	— liver
Gastro	— stomach	Angio	— a duct
Entro	— small bowel	Haemangio	— a blood vessel
Chole	— bile	Lymphangio	— a lymph vessel
Col	— colon	Phleb	— a vein
Proct	— rectum	Arteri	— artery
Cyst	— bladder	Thromb	— a clot
Ileo	— ileum	Colp	— vagina
Jejuno	— jejunum	Mast ·	— breast
Nephr	— kidney	Mammo	
Diverticul	— diverticulum	Pyelo	— renal pelvis
Myo	— muscle		

E.g. most others are obvious from everyday usage

Chol—angio—gram	— an x-ray of the bile ducts.
Chole—cysto—gram	— an x-ray of the gall bladder.
Pan—procto—colectomy	— excision of the whole rectum and colon.
Thromb—endarter—ectomy	— excision of a clot and lining of the artery.
Gastro—jejun—ostomy	— the formation of a new opening between stomach and jejunum.

17
Inflammation and Wound Healing

Inflammation is the reaction of living tissue to trauma. Trauma is not necessarily infection, but can be a physical agent such as heat, cold, a wound, or x-ray; or it can be chemical, as in burns due to carbolic or phosphorus; or it can be due to infection. The process of inflammation is part of the body's defence mechanism and is concerned with the bringing of the body's defences to bear at the point of injury. It is marked by the classical five signs of

1. Heat
2. Pain
3. Redness
4. Swelling
5. Loss of function

The first thing that is seen following injury is that there is a dilation of the vessels of the skin. This leads to redness of the part and with the increased blood flow through the skin the part becomes warm, and serum oozes out into the surrounding tissues. The serum carries with it antibodies for defence against micro-organisms and also white cells to attack and overcome infection, or to ingest foreign materials. This exudation of fluid and cells into the area surrounding the injury produces the swelling and the combination of swelling and congestion of the part is often what causes the pain rather than the actual injury itself. When a part is painful and inflamed, function is lost and the part is held at rest. This aids in the localisation of the injury or infection.

These changes of inflammation are seen most easily in the skin and can be demonstrated following a simple scratch with a pin and in a condition such as a septic finger where all are shown to good advantage. They occur, however, in all the tissues of the body, although they may be less obvious elsewhere. These same changes of inflammation are essential for the process of wound healing, for after all, a wound is simply trauma to the body and the body's reaction is always the same.

Wounds may be of many types – they may be clean or dirty, ragged and lacerated or sharp and incised, but in surgery we are considering mostly the surgical incision which is a clean, incised wound, and consideration of the healing of this wound will serve to illustrate the healing of all injuries with loss of tissue or damage of tissue.

Following the wound, the process of inflammation develops on both sides of the cut surface, there is an increase in the blood flow to the part, redness, swelling and an out-pouring of blood plasma and white cells into the gap between the edges of the wound. This fills up the space and clots, sticking the wound edges together. Then blood vessels and new tissue grow in from each side and 'darn' the wound together. At this stage the wound is healed, sound and bright red in appearance due to the presence of the capillaries. Over the next few months the scar tissue contracts and tightens, sealing the wound edges more firmly together and so the scar takes on a typical pure white appearance of mature fibrous tissue. While these changes are occurring in the depth of the wound the epithelium on the surface grows across to establish continuity.

In the surgical incision where the wound is stitched together the tissues are placed in close approximation and so there is little distance to be covered in the healing process, and healing is rapid. If, however, the wound edges are wide apart, or if there is much loss of tissue, then the whole of this gap has to be filled with the growing capillaries and fibrous tissue. This takes, of course, a very much longer time. This type of healing is best seen in an ulcer where the base of the ulcer becomes like red velvet, covered with a soft red mass of new blood vessels, which slowly build up until the whole gap of the wound is filled and it lies flush with the surrounding surface. When it reaches this stage the epithelium from the edge of the ulcer grows across and eventually covers the surface. When this process matures the contraction of the fibrous tissue pulls the skin surface down and so gives rise to a depressed scar.

It is obvious from this that the more closely we can approximate the wound edges the quicker and sounder will be the healing and the stronger the resulting scar, with the minimum deformity.

The outcome of inflammation can be either resolution, in which the whole process subsides with no trace that any injury has ever occurred.

This can only happen where there has been minimal tissue damage. If tissue damage has been marked then the result of inflammation is repair and the formation of scar tissue, as in the wound healing just described. In the case of infection, then the result of inflammatory reaction can be progression to suppuration, i.e. the formation of pus. When infection gains an entry it is surrounded immediately by the inflammatory reaction and fluid and white cells are poured into the area. If the infection is severe then there will be death of the tissues affected and at the same time there will be death of large numbers of bacteria destroyed by the antibodies in the serum and white cells, and so a plug of dead tissue develops. This is called a slough. Around this slough there is the formation of pus. Pus is merely fluid which contains dead bacteria and white cells, both dead and alive. Pus has powerful liquifying properties and so when a slough develops surrounded by pus it erodes the overlying tissues and presents on the surface of the body where it discharges, leaving a hole. This slough surrounded by pus is what we call an abcess. When it discharges on to the surface of the body it leaves a cavity which is an ulcer. This formation of pus and discharge on to the skin assumes that the body has been able to overcome the infection. If, however, the infection is not localised by the inflammatory reaction, then spread occurs. Spread of infection can occur in the tissue spaces between the cells when it is known as a cellulitis. This is most likely to occur in infections with the streptococcus, or spread can occur via the lymphatic pathways to give an infection of the lymphatics and lymphangitis. If the infection spreads by the lymphatics it will eventually reach the related lymphatic glands. These are rather like large filters, which filter out impurities. The infection tends to be trapped here and may go on to form suppuration in the gland with secondary abcesses. In the worst possible outcome, the infection may spread to the blood stream, giving rise to septicaemia. This is a very severe condition in which the patient becomes very toxic and it often proves fatal. Occasionally thrombosis (i.e. clotting) of the vessels occurs in the abcess wall related to the pus and little bits of septic blood clot may break off and travel in the blood stream as emboli; this is known as pyemia, and wherever these little blood clots become stuck within the body they form new abscesses, called metastatic abscesses. This also is a very severe and often fatal condition.

It will be seen, therefore, that inflammation is one of the essential processes of defence of the body against trauma. Occasionally, however, the inflammatory response is out of all proportion to the degree of trauma and in these cases it is the inflammation which renders the patient ill, rather than the actual process which stimulates it. For instance, in a sprained ankle the sprain itself is often minimal and what causes the pain and discomfort to the patient is the gross swelling and inflammatory response occurring due to the injury. Similarly, in infections of the testis or the epididymus, it is often the inflammatory response accompanying the infection which causes the patient's pain and discomfort. In other conditions, such as rheumatoid arthritis, it is the inflammatory response in the joints which gives the severe crippling changes rather than the stimulus to the inflammation. In these cases, we sometimes wish to stop the inflammatory response. This can be done by means of drugs derived from the adrenal cortex, such as cortisone, hydrocortisone or any of its derivatives. It can also be eased by drugs of the butazolidine type. These, however, although they may be beneficial in the diseases mentioned, are dangerous as they also reduce the body's reaction to infection. Any patient who is on cortisone or its derivatives is more prone to intermittent infection than a normal person and any infection occurring should be treated immediately with large doses of broad spectrum antibiotics.

Abscesses also give rise to systemic upset as well as the local changes that occur. The patient feels ill and often has a raised temperature and pulse rate, the appetite is spoiled, the patient is thirsty and is often constipated. All of these are signs of a severely ill patient.

If there is a cavity containing a lot of pus in the body, the temperature often swings daily to a high level and this is fairly typical of suppuration. In these instances the patient may be so ill that it becomes essential to drain the abscess, rather than to wait for it to erode its way to the surface itself. However, an abscess must not be incised and drained too soon, because if it is not well localised an incision into it may merely serve to spread the infection. The treatment of all abscesses, no matter the situation on the body, is an incision into them and drainage of the contained pus. This is immediately followed by a dramatic improvement in the patient's condition, the temperature falls to normal, the patient feels much better, the appetite returns and healing occurs by repair and fibrosis more or less rapidly, depending on the size of the cavity which is left.

A wound infection is merely a specialised form of abscess, in which infection occurs in the healing wound. The introduction of sepsis most commonly occurs in the theatre at the time the wound is made. When the wound is stitched up the infection is sealed in the depths of the wound often in the presence of blood clot which forms a perfect culture medium in which the organisms may multiply. Pus forms in the depths of the wound, the patient becomes ill with a raised or swinging temperature, and toxic, and often it is some considerable time before evidence occurs at the surface of the wound. The treatment of this, however, is no different from that of an abscess anywhere else. Once the infection is localised, it should be drained. In the case of a wound this is often made simple because the wound has already been made and all that is required is to remove one or two stitches in the neighbourhood of the abscess and gently separate the wound edges with a pair of sinus forceps to allow the pus to escape. Once again this is usually followed by a dramatic improvement in the patient's condition.

Most surgical incisions are repaired in layers, each layer of the tissues, muscle fascia, peritoneum and skin being separately sutured. In general the deeper layers, where stitches are going to be permanent and buried, are repaired with absorbable suture material such as catgut, while the skin is repaired with unabsorbable material such as nylon or silk. If, however, the tissue has a poor blood supply, such as tendon, or the layer of fibrous tissue covering muscles then unabsorbable sutures are used since healing in these tissues may take many weeks. The materials used may be nylon or terylene, silk or linen, or in some cases stainless steel wire. These give a very sound repair but it is essential when unabsorbable sutures are being used that no infection must be present since any trace of sepsis will cause these materials to be extruded as foreign bodies and the wound will continue to discharge until all the foreign material has been released.

18
Shock and Haemorrhage

Shock is due to a fall in blood pressure. This can be due to bleeding or to dilation of the arteries and veins caused by nervous stimulation.

Shock is characterised by a fall in the blood pressure coupled with a rise in pulse rate, the patient is anxious, restless, sweating, thirsty and pale, the skin feels cold and clammy.

In haemorrhagic shock (shock due to bleeding) the treatment is to replace the blood loss. In neurogenic shock (due to nervous causes) where there has been no blood loss, sometimes blood is used to quickly restore the blood pressure. There is no place in modern medicine for the use of plasma, either for the treatment of shock or for replacing protein in the blood, the risk of infective hepatitis is much too high, and it is now superceded by synthetic substances such as Macrodex. Drugs which close the blood vessels can also be used.

Blood transfusion is indicated mainly to replace the blood loss due to haemorrhage. It is, however, used to correct gross anaemia and in particular to bring the haemoglobin level towards normal if the patient is going to require surgery. Surgery for any condition is contraindicated with a haemoglobin below 80%. Blood transfusion, however, is not without its dangers. These may be listed as follows:

1. Transfusion reaction, due to incompatible blood
2. Allergic and pyrogenic reactions (collapse with high fever)
3. The risk of infection.
4. The dangers common to all intravenous infusions.

The biggest danger of all is the risk of giving incompatible blood. Blood for transfusion into a patient must be matched against the patient's own blood. There are many factors which require to be matched, but in general only two groups are regularly checked. This is the ABO blood group of patient and donor, and the Rhesus (Rh) factor. However, even assuming that the AB group is correctly matched and the Rh factor, it is still possible for the blood to react unfavourably. Therefore all patients should have their blood cross-matched with the donor blood immediately before transfusion.

There are four blood groups —

Group A
Group B
Group AB
Group O

When incompatible blood is given the patient develops a transfusion reaction. The temperature usually rises to a high level, the patient becomes sweaty, shivery, and collapsed. The blood pressure falls and jaundice often develops. The kidneys may fail to produce urine (anuria) and death may occur.

It is rare for blood to be mis-matched in the laboratory and most commonly the giving of incompatible blood is due to a mistake at ward level. It is absolutely imperative that when setting up a bottle of blood intravenously the patient's name and address on the casesheet should be checked against the name and address on the bottle of blood. The form showing the blood group and Rh factor on the patient's notes should be checked against that on the bottle of blood and only if all agree should the blood be given. It is important to remember that any substance given intravenously is effective almost instantaneously. This applies equally to drugs and to all intravenous infusions, and any substance given intravenously is gone beyond recall. Therefore the utmost care should be taken in checking everything before it is given by the intravenous route.

All intravenous infusions are prone to give rise to certain complications. These may be listed as follows.

1. Thrombophlebitis (painful clotting) of the vein used for the infusion.
2. Allergic and pyrogenic reactions due to chemicals derived from the giving sets of bottles.
3. The risk of infection.
4. Allergic reactions to the substance being infused.
5. The administration of too much fluid which in the elderly patient may precipitate congestive cardiac failure, the ageing heart being unable to cope with the additional load being pushed on the right side of the heart.

Most of these are the concern of the doctor in charge of the patient, but air embolism occurs when the bottle is allowed to run through and this is one situation where the nurse should be constantly on the look out during her normal ward duties, to makes sure that the bottles are changed and a fresh bottle put up before the fluid has run through. To this end it is always a good principle to have the next bottle required at the end of the patient's bed, so that as soon as the bottle is finished it can be changed without the infusion being switched off, which carries the risk of thrombosis in the vein and the necessity of discontinuing the infusion.

Apart from blood, intravenous therapy is used to replace fluid, electrolytes and nutritional substances which the patient requires urgently. Generally speaking fluid, electrolytes, and food are all taken best via the alimentary canal and intravenous therapy is no substitute for normal feeding. However, in many instances an infusion is needed because

1. The patient is unable to take fluid by mouth
2. Is unable to absorb nutrition given by mouth either because he is on naso-gastric suction, or because the bowel is paralysed as in an ileus, or because there are fistulae (leaks) which drain away intestinal contents.
3. There may be excessive loss of fluid and electrolytes from the body as in diarrhoea or vomiting.

As far as fluid is concerned, the maintenance of an intake and output chart is of the utmost importance and gives perhaps the best guide to the patient's requirements, as one day's output determines the next day's intake.

Rather than maintaining a battery of solutions for intravenous use, the principle in most hospitals is to have a certain number of basic solutions to which additions can be made. These usually involve solutions of isotonic sugar, such as 5% dextrose and distilled water, solutions of normal saline either with or without glucose, and solutions of sugar such as fructose or alcohol, and solutions of amino acids. To the basic electrolyte solutions can be added potassium in the form of potassium chloride, additional glucose or fructose, bicarbonate to correct the patient's acid base balance, manitol to produce a diuresis in the patient who is passing little urine, or ammonium chloride, again to correct alkalosis. As far as intravenous feeding is concerned, the patient should have a minimum of 50 Gm of protein a day, plus 2000–3000 Calories, and the doctor in charge requires to prepare a regime including fats, sugars and amino acids to provide this amount without an excessive amount of fluid.

NOTES

APPROXIMATE DAILY ADULT REQUIREMENTS

Water Intake .... 2,000 ml (70 fl. ozs.)	
Urine Output .... 800 ml. (28 fl. ozs.)	Safe Minima
Sodium Chloride .... 4·5 grams	
Potassium Chloride .... 2·0 grams	

COMPOSITION OF INTRAVENOUS FLUIDS

DESCRIPTION	CONTENT	
	WATER	SOLUTE
Normal Saline Solution (Isotonic)		
1 Pint (20 fl. ozs.)	568 ml.	Sodium Chloride 5 grams
1 Litre	1,000 ml.	" 9 grams
5% Glucose Solution (Isotonic)		
1 Pint (20 fl. ozs.)	568 ml.	Glucose 28 grams
1 Litre	1,000 ml.	" 50 grams
10% Glucose Solution (Isotonic)		
1 Pint (20 fl. ozs.)	568 ml.	Glucose 56 grams
1 Litre	1,000 ml.	" 100 grams

CONVERSION VALUES

1 fl. oz	= 28·5ml.	1 litre	= 35 fl. ozs.
1 pint	= 568ml.	1 ml.	= 17 minims
1 oz.	= 28 grams	1 gram	= 15·5 grains.

GLASGOW ROYAL INFIRMARY — **DAY CHART**

SURNAME (Block Letters)	FIRST NAMES	DATE	WARD	AGE	UNIT NUMBER

TIME	INTAKE				OUTPUT				NOTES
	WATER				WATER				
	ORAL	RECTAL	INTRAVENOUS	TOTAL	URINE	GASTRIC CONTENTS	FISTULA	TOTAL	
8									
9									
10									
11									
12									
1									
2									
3									
4									
5									
6									
7									
TOTAL									

19
Varicose Veins and Ulcers

Varicose Veins

Varicose veins are one of the penalties man pays for walking upright. It is quite unknown in any other animal. The typical varicose vein is too well known to need description. Basically it is a dilation and increased tortuosity of the superficial veins of the lower limb. Two factors are at work. One is a defect of the valves allowing the weight of the column of blood from the rest of the body to press down into the veins of the legs. This high pressure of blood causes the dilation and tortuosity which in turn destroys further valves.

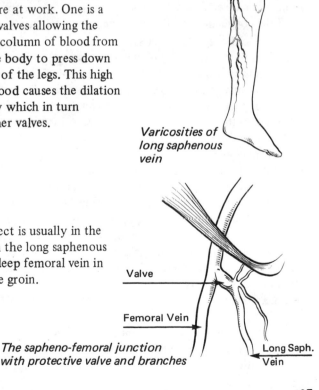

Varicosities of long saphenous vein

The basic defect is usually in the valve between the long saphenous vein and the deep femoral vein in the fold of the groin.

Valve

Femoral Vein

The sapheno-femoral junction with protective valve and branches

Long Saph. Vein

As a general rule varicose veins are common in people whose jobs involve long periods of standing but they can also be precipitated by increases in intra-abdominal pressure such as pregnancy, ovarian cysts and large abdominal tumours. Occasionally they may follow deep venous thrombosis in the leg where the deep veins become blocked with clot and the total blood from the deep veins has to be diverted to the superficial system. The treatment of varicose veins aims at obliterating the vein or disconnecting it from the high pressure venous blood which is distending it. Needless to say, varicose veins must not be treated if the deep vein of the leg is blocked. Treatment may be surgical which usually consists of dividing the long saphenous vein at the groin and removing the vein by stripping it out from the ankle to the groin. However, the same effect may be achieved by multiple ligation at the groin, the ankle and above and below the knee which are the sites at which the connections to the deep vein most commonly occur. The other vein in the leg, the short saphenous which runs from the outside of the foot to the back of the knee may also be involved and treatment here again is by ligation at the knee and stripping out the vein.

Non-operative treatment consists of injections. These can be used for small insignificant veins to achieve a cosmetic result but recently are being used in the treatment of fully developed varicose veins to produce obliteration of the vein at the sites where connection to the deep vein occurs. Pressure is then put on the vein by means of sponge rubber and a firm bandage applied. These bandages are kept in place for six weeks and this is an essential part of the treatment. During this time they are looked at every two weeks and further injection given if necessary. Sometimes, however, operation is not feasible either because of the patient's general condition or because a previous operation has failed. In these cases only palliative treatment is possible. This is carried out by means of compression bandaging either by means of a crepe bandage or more commonly by use of an elastic stocking. The elastic stockings to be effective are always thick, heavy and are cosmetically unappealing as well as being extremely hot and unpleasant in summer. The treatment of varicose veins by elastic stockings should only be where the veins are unsuitable for surgery or for injection.

Varicose Ulcers

Varicose ulceration occurs in patients who have venous stasis in the legs usually associated with varicose veins. The venous return from the legs is slow and venous blood tends to pool round the ankles. The skin becomes water logged and unhealthy. This is often first manifested by an itchiness and irritation of the skin and often a scaly eruption to give a dermatitis. Through scratching this or through an injury in this unhealthy skin, the skin breaks down to form a small ulcer. This is slow to heal and it often enlarges to a considerable size before healing commences. These ulcers often heal, only to break down again, and this cycle may continue for many years. Very rarely the irritation of this chronic ulceration may lead to the development of a malignant tumour.

The treatment of these ulcers is many and varied. All will heal with bed rest and elevation of the limb to improve the circulation. However, it is not feasible for the average person to spend many weeks in bed to heal the ulcer. An attempt to heal the ulcer with the patient ambulant is made by applying some firm support technique. This may be in the form of the medicated semi-rigid bandage such as Unna's paste or viscopaste or maybe by means of a non-elastic rigid stocking. This is often used in conjunction with physiotherapy. There is massage given to the edge of the ulcer to stimulate it, a medicated dressing is cut and applied to the ulcer base and the special bandage applied over this. This treatment is known as the Bisgaard treatment. In many instances, however, surgery is eventually required for healing of the ulcer. Surgery is aimed at the underlying venous stasis and may consist of treatment of the co-existing varicose veins or a more direct attack on the veins underlying the ulcer which are divided. This usually enables the ulcer to heal. If, however, the healing is slow and the ulcer is large, healing can be accelerated by the application of a split skin graft taken from the thigh to the surface of the ulcer. With varicose veins being treated more commonly nowadays in their early stages, it is to be hoped that the incidence of venous or stasis ulcer will become progressively less.

20
The Breast

In humans there are normally two developed breasts in the female. These lie over the front of the chest stretching from the clavicle to the sixth rib and from the edge of the sternum to the level of the front of the axilla. A small piece of breast tissue lies in the axilla behind the anterior fold and is known as the axillary tail. Occasionally in the male the breasts also develop.

The lymph drainage of the breasts is in all directions like the spokes of a wheel the most important radiating to the axilla where enlarged glands are commonly found.

Diseases of the Breast.

The diseases of the breast that the surgeon is called on to deal with are those due to physical abnormality, to abcess formation and to tumours, simple and malignant. These will be dealt with separately.

Congenital Malformations

The absence of breasts or nipples is rare, but quite frequently extra nipples or extra mammary tissue occur in the so-called milk line extending from the axilla to the groin. Normally these give rise to no upset but occasionally, during pregnancy, accessory or supernumery breasts may develop along with the normal breasts and give rise to discomfort and unsightliness. Treatment is by simple excision of the accessory tissue.

Mammary Hypertrophy

The breasts normally start developing to their adult size at the time of puberty and by the late teens, the breasts have usually assumed their adult shape and form, and cease growth. Occasionally, however, the breasts may continue to grow and become extremely large, heavy and uncomfortable. This is known as simple hypertrophy of the breast. This condition in the past used to be dealt with by amputation of the breasts as they caused so much discomfort and were thought to be prone to malignant change. Nowadays the plastic surgeon reduces the size of the breasts to a more normal acceptable size. The operation is known as reduction Mammoplasty. Occasionally, and only for cosmetic reasons, breasts which are rather small may be increased in size by the opposite type of technique known as an augmentation Mammoplasty.

Infections

Infections can affect the breast as any other tissue of the body. There are few which require surgical treatment. In the past, tuberculosis occasionally affected the breast and required mastectomy. Syphilis can also affect the breast either in its primary or in its more advanced forms. The commonest infection however, is a simple pyogenic infection occurring during lactation. When the breasts are full and engorged with milk they form an ideal culture medium for bacteria and these gain access to the breast during suckling via cracks in the nipples. This leads to a cellulitis of the breast which if not quickly controlled by antibiotics goes on to abscess formation. Surgical treatment is to drain the abscess. An incision is made into the abscess and the fibrous tissue splitting it up into segments broken down with the finger and free drainage established. A drain is usually inserted through a dependant part of the breast so that gravity aids the drainage of pus. Healing is remarkably rapid. When infection develops in the breast the baby must be weaned and lactation suppressed by drugs.

Simple Tumours of the Breast

Any simple tumour can occur in the breast but only one is of any significance. This is the tumour known as fibroadenoma. There is a diffuse form of this condition called fibroadenosis. In this condition both the fibrous tissue and the glandular tissue of the breast enlarge and the breasts become irregular and shotty with many little nodules palpable throughout the breast. This is a very common condition and develops in the late teens and is prominent in the twenties and thirties. The breasts tend to become painful at the time of the periods when there is water retention, and the breasts normally swell slightly at this time. This part of the condition is known as premenstrual tension. Occasionally, one of these nodules may enlarge progressively to form a discrete lump in the breast, a fibroadenoma. This may also be painful at period times but is usually the size of it which draws it to the patient's notice. The condition is simple and is treated by excision of the lump. In the case of the diffuse disease, surgery is rarely required. Treatment is to reassure

131

the patient, to advise on a well fitting bra and perhaps the use of a diuretic for the seven days before the period to reduce the water retention. However, there is rarely the patient in whom the breasts are so painful at period times that a simple mastectomy is required.

Another less common tumour is the duct papilloma. This is a small wart which grows in the ducts of the breast near the nipple and leads to a blood stained discharge from the nipple. On examination of the breast there are no palpable lumps but pressing on the affected quadrant, blood can be expressed from the nipple. Treatment of this condition is a wedge excision of the part of the breast containing the wart.

Malignant Tumours of the Breast

The only malignant tumour of the breast of any significance is cancer. This occurs in 4% of all women. It is an extremely malignant tumour but by lying in a fairly accessible part of the body, if it is diagnosed early, the chances of "cure" are very good. Unfortunately, the disease does not produce dramatic symptoms. It starts with a small painless lump in the breast which is usually only noticed by chance during bathing. The disease spreads through the overlying tissues to perhaps involve the skin of the breast. It spreads in the lymphatics to affect the lymph glands usually in the axilla of the same side, perhaps those in the neck, in the mediastinum beside the lungs and even down into the abdomen. It also spreads in the blood stream to affect primarily

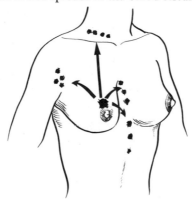

Lymphatic spread from carcinoma of breast

the bones, especially those in the lumbar spine. We divide cancer of the breast, clinically into four stages.

1. The first stage is where the lump is small and confined to the breast.
2. The second stage is where there are glands palpable in the axilla.
3. The third stage is where the skin of the breast is ulcerated and the tumour is stuck to the deep muscles of the chest wall.
4. The fourth stage is where distant spread has occurred to organs other than the breast.

The stage the patient is in when first seen greatly influences their chance of survival. The patient whose tumour is in stage one has a 70% chance of being alive and well in five years. The patient in stage two on the other hand has only a 50% chance of being alive and well at the end of five years. In stage three the chances are only about 20% while all patients in stage four will be dead within twelve months of being seen. It is obviously of great importance to diagnose these tumours early and in this connection the education of the public has a great part to play. Women over the age of 40 should be encouraged to examine their breasts regularly while bathing to look for any sign of a lump. The

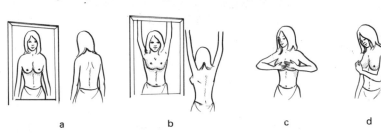

a   b   c   d

Self examination of breast.
a) Observation of breasts in mirror
b) Observation of breasts with arms elevated
*   noting levels of nipples and shape*
c) Palpation of breasts with flat of hand
d) Palpation of breasts with finger and thumb

disease can occur in any age but is more common in the 40/60 age group.

The treatment of cancer of the breast depends upon the stage at which the disease is diagnosed. The treatments are many and varied but basically, they involve excision of the tumour and the surrounding breast and/or radiotherapy. Removal of the breast may be of the breast tissue alone, when it is known as a simple mastectomy, or it may involve removal of the breast, the underlying muscles and the glands enlarged in the axilla, when it is known as a radical mastectomy. There

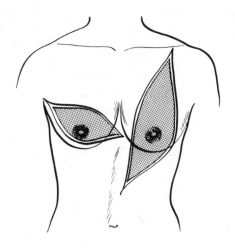

Incisions used for mastectomy

are many and varied other varieties of mastectomy which are modifications of these two basic types. Radiotherapy can be given alone or can be given after operation to destroy any cancer cells that have been left by the surgeon. Generally speaking if the disease is in stage one or stage two then mastectomy is carried out followed by radiotherapy, the type of mastectomy depending on the surgeon's personal preference. In stage three usually radiotherapy alone is given, although for cosmetic reasons some form of palliative removal of the tumour may be necessary to prevent ulceration of the skin. In stage four there is rarely any point in treating the primary lesion since the tumour is widely disseminated, but again, for cosmetic purposes, radiotherapy or surgery may be required. Some tumours of the breast are dependent on the circulating level of female sex hormones. This tends to be the case in tumours occurring in women before the menopause and, in these cases, it is reasonable to remove the ovaries as these are the prime source of female sex hormones. It is therefore fairly standard in the patient who is pre-menopausal or up to five years after the menopause to have an oophorectomy (removal of ovaries) carried out following treatment of the primary lesion. However, this can be left and carried out if signs of metastases develop — this again depends on the preference of the surgeon. If removal of the ovaries produces some benefit then further endocrine procedures can be carried out to gain further palliation. Other sources of the female sex hormone are the adrenal glands and so adrenalectomy can be carried out. In some centres, however, an alternative treatment is removal of the pituitary gland. Both of these procedures means that the patient requires to be put on a maintenance dose of Cortisone for the rest of her life. Operative adrenalectomy is now becoming less common because the same effect can be achieved by the giving of large doses of steroids — this is known as medical adrenalectomy. Another type of hormone treatment is to administer male sex hormones to the patient. This used to be in the form of testosterone implants under the skin but this led to a lot of side effects which were upsetting. The female form tended to change towards a male form but, more particularly, the patient developed a beard and a moustache, which was most upsetting. Nowadays steroids are available which have the same effect but without side effects.

These are known as anabolic steroids and form another useful method of treatment in cancer of the breast.

Quite apart from treatment of the primary lesion, radiotherapy has a large part to play in the treatment of metastases. These most commonly affect the spine and give rise to severe pain and collapse of the vertebrae. They may also affect the bones of the pelvis and the thigh and occasionally lead to fracture of the femur. Radiotherapy to these bony metastases can often give considerable pain relief and give the patient much comfort. There are also available drugs which depress tumour growth and these are called cytotoxic drugs. It will be seen that there are many and varied treatments of cancer of the breast and, in spite of the intensive research that has gone into this disease for many generations, there is still no one strict line of treatment and any or all of these methods of treatment can be used together in combination or one after another. The strict order will depend on the hospital and the particular surgeon concerned.

The patient who has to have a mastectomy performed requires very careful psychological care as she experiences fears of mutilation, loss of femininity or becoming something of an oddity as a result of this operation. As some will also be experiencing the menopause it can make the situation particularly trying, so constant reassurance and sympathetic handling are essential.

Physical preparation will include axillary and chest shave. A skin graft is occasionally required, so the thigh and pubic area should be prepared in addition.

In the post-operative care of this patient the wound requires special care. A drain may be in position and if it is attached to a suction machine the pressure should not rise above two centimetres of mercury. The drain should be left in position for two to five days and some blood, but mainly serous fluid, may be drained. This drain prevents the fluid from collecting under the skin and thus aids healing. The patient's sutures would be removed after eight to ten days but care would be taken to observe that the wound edges were healthy. Once the wound is healed the patient should be supplied with an adequate prosthesis. This should be fitted before dismissal to minimise the psychological effect of the operation, but if the wound is too tender the bra could be padded with cottonwool until the prosthesis can be worn.

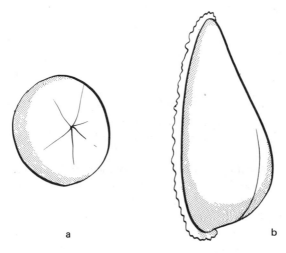

Mammary prostheses
a) Malpro — "bird-seed" prosthesis
b) Tru-form — liquid filled prosthesis

There are several types of prosthesis made of pads filled with plastic seed, foam rubber, fluid or air, and the one most suited to the patient's need should be ordered. The modern fluid filled bra can be worn even under bikini type swimwear and although expensive is a useful aid in restoring the patient's confidence.

The patient should have the arm on the effected side carefully supported on pillows and the nurse should observe it for any swelling. Movements of the hand and elbow joint should be encouraged immediately after operation. Exercises are essential to prevent the development of shoulder joint deformities and will be commenced after specific orders from the surgeon. These may consist of ordinary tasks such as brushing and combing her hair, washing or attempting to manage back fastenings on clothing. She will be allowed up to sit probably on the first post-operative day. She may experience a slight upset in balance but the nurse should encourage her to hold an upright posture.

The nurse must observe the patient's reaction to the operation. Individuals react in different ways to stressful situations and this may be demonstrated by frequent bouts of crying, anger, or withdrawal from others. Some patients put a brave face on things while in hospital but become depressed on return home. The nurse must be aware of the variety of reactions which can be expected and be kindly and understanding in her attitude.

The patient should be advised and encouraged to return to normal living as soon as possible after dismissal. Recommencement of social life should be assumed but the patient should be observed for depressive periods. She will require a great deal of support from her husband, if married, and her family.

As already mentioned patients may have an operation on the breast followed by radiotherapy treatment. This is not commenced until the patient's skin is healed and since the patient's resistance to infection may be reduced by this treatment she should be instructed to steer clear of people who have colds. The patient's skin while undergoing radiotherapy treatment should not have any ointment on it and the area involved should not be washed during the treatment. The patient may have a local reaction rather like bad sunburn to this treatment. She may have periods of nausea, vomiting, may lose her appetite or feel a little unwell while having the treatment.

On return home the patient may have periods of tiredness and lack of energy and she will require a period of convalescence before resuming work and should return to the hospital for regular checks.

21
The Thorax

Anatomy

The thorax or chest is that part of the body enclosed by the ribs and separated from the abdomen by the diaphragm. It contains the two lungs which are separated by a partition known as the mediastinum. This partition contains the heart, great vessels, oesophagus and thymus gland. Each lung is encased in a membrane known as the pleura and this is reflected at the root of the lung to line the corresponding half of the chest. Thus a potential space is present between chest wall and lung lined on both sides by pleura. This is known as the pleural space. The lungs are like elastic sponges and outwith the body are collapsed. During inspiration when the rib cage expands and the diaphragm descends a negative pressure (or suction) develops in the pleural space and the lung expands to fill the space drawing in air through the trachea as it does so. When inspiration stops and the muscles relax the elasticity of the lung makes it collapse pushing the air back out again so giving expiration. This sequence of events repeated continually constitutes breathing and is an automatic involuntary mechanism. It can, however, be modified by voluntary control.

Surgery on the Chest

With the development of modern anaesthesia and resuscitative techniques, the chest which was once a barrier to the surgeon is now a fairly routine site for surgery. The chest requires to be opened for-

1 Injuries of the chest
2 Diseases of the lung
3 Diseases of the heart and great vessels in the chest
4 Diseases of the oesophagus

Heart disease will be discussed elsewhere and the oesophagus has been discussed in a separate chapter.

Chest injuries may be closed or open. A closed chest injury is one in which communication between the pleural cavity and the outside air has not occurred. It is becoming extremely common in the form of

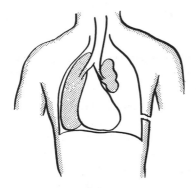

Open pneumothorax with mediastinal shift.

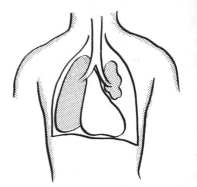

Closed pneumothorax

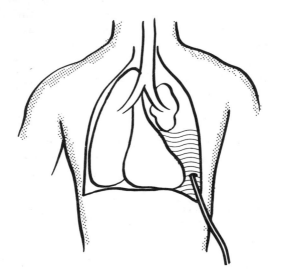

Haemopneumothorax with drainage.

crushed chest which occurs in motor accidents. There are multiple broken ribs with inability of that part of the chest to expand, while damage to the underlying lung may cause bleeding into the lung or into the pleural cavity (haemothorax). Any fluid in the chest whether blood, pus, or serum causes collapse of the underlying lung and should be drained. Drains for fluid will be placed in the lower chest for dependent drainage while to remove air they are placed at the upper part of the chest. Damage to the lung may also allow the escape of air into the pleural cavity (pneumothorax) again with collapse of the underlying lung. Occasionally the lung damage allows air to be drawn into the pleural cavity with each inspiration so that the pressure steadily rises. This results in displacement of the mediastinum to the opposite side with collapse of the opposite lung. This is called tension pneumothorax and is quickly fatal if not relieved.

The treatment of these closed chest injuries is to establish adequate respiration. This will involve draining fluid or air from the pleural cavity to allow the lung to re-expand, intensive physiotherapy, adequate sedation for pain relief and perhaps positive pressure ventilation to expand the lung from within. A check on the adequacy of respiration can be achieved by measuring the amounts of oxygen, carbon dioxide and acidity in arterial blood, this is known as "doing the blood gases",

Open chest injuries are commonly due to a penetrating wound such as stabbing. A pneumothorax is present and the underlying lung may have been damaged with bleeding (haemopneumothorax). The risk of infection is high. The principles of treatment are the same as for closed injuries. The wound is excised and closed with drainage instituted to allow the lung to expand.

Diseases of the lung which require surgery are tuberculosis, cancer, simple tumours of the lung, or infections, such as bronchiectasis. The whole lung may be removed in the operation (pneumonectomy) or only a portion of the lung (lobectomy).

Tuberculosis

Tuberculosis is much less common today than in the past but may still call for surgical treatment. This may be a form of treatment designed to collapse the portion of the lung affected by the tuberculosis and so allow it to rest. This can be by the introduction of an artificial

141

pneumothorax or an artificial pneumo-peritoneum. These are temporary measures. If more permanent collapse of the lung is required then operation is carried out to remove the overlying ribs and allow the soft tissue to press in and collapse the underlying lung. This operation is known as thoracoplasty. However, with effective anti-tuberculous drugs now available the requirements for these operations are becoming less and at the same time the risk of spread of the disease due to surgery is also less and surgical treatment has therefore tended to be more aggressive and it is now feasible to excise the affected portions of lung (lobectomy).

Tumours of the lung

Sometimes simple tumours of the lung occur, which give rise to severe symptoms and the treatment in these conditions is to excise the affected portion of lung. However, one of the steadily increasing diseases of our age is cancer of the lung. If this disease is diagnosed early and if the patient is fit, then the treatment is operative. However, it must be remembered that the patient must be left with sufficient pulmonary function to allow a normal life. There is little point in excising a tumour of lung if the patient is left so breathless that he is unable to move out of bed.

For this reason the pulmonary function must be carefully assessed and it is unusual to carry out operation in patients over fifty-five years of age. This tumour of lung has a close tie-up with cigarette-smoking and, apart from the tumour, cigarette-smoking does lead to chronic bronchitis which diminishes the function of the remaining lung and these patients are often unsuitable for chest surgery. However, it is the treatment of choice if it is at all feasible. The tumour is removed, with the affected portion of lung and this often requires a pneumonectomy. In addition the glands in the mediastinum to which the tumour will spread are removed.

Bronchiectasis

This is a disease in which there is chronic abscess formation in the walls of the bronchi. The patient has a chronic cough and purulent sputum. If the disease is localised to one area of the lung then it is feasible to carry out resection of this portion of the lung and eradicate the septic focus, as otherwise it leads to chronic ill health and premature death. Operation may be required for other infective conditions of the chest. If there is pus in the chest (pyothorax) this will require to be drained also, or perhaps, if it is localised, excision of the abscess and surrounding lung.

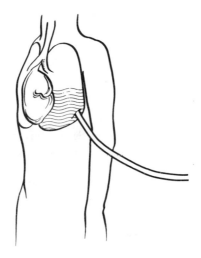

Chest drainage

Surgery inside the chest always requires drainage of the chest thereafter and this requires the use of a waterseal drain. Since the function of the lungs depends on the development of a negative pressure of suction within the pleural cavity as the chest is expanded, then any communication of the pleural cavity with the outside air causes the lung to collapse and inhibits respiration. Thus, to drain the chest, the drain cannot be connected to any system where air might enter the chest. It is therefore connected to a bottle on the floor containing water plus some antiseptic. Air from the pleural cavity can thus bubble through the water and escape while pus, blood or other fluids can drain freely into the water, but air is unable to re-enter the pleural cavity. This will be seen more clearly in the following diagram.

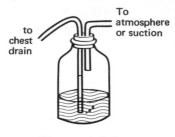

to
chest
drain

To
atmosphere
or suction

Water seal drain

It is obvious that no part of the system should be disconnected
lest air enter the chest. If the bottle requires to be emptied or change
then two large pressure forceps should be placed on the drain close to
the patient. A skilled nurse should always be made responsible for the
care of a chest drainage system. The chest drain is left in the chest until
drainage has ceased or until the lung has completely expanded. Removal
of the chest drain entails the risk of air entering the chest as the tube is
withdrawn. When removing a chest drain, therefore, the patient should be
instructed to expire and "hold it" as the drain is pulled out in a quick
movement and an occlusive dressing applied over the drainage site.

22
Head Injuries

The patient who has sustained a head injury may be conscious or unconscious on admission. It is essential, particularly in the unconscious patient, that other injuries are not overlooked and a detailed examination of the whole patient carried out. Investigation should include examination of the nervous system to establish a base line of conscious level and any paralysis as any change in these is important. X-ray of the skull may be carried out but is not of particular help as fractures of the skull themselves are not of importance only the effects they produce by damage to nerve, brain, or by haemorrhage. Also the fractures which produce damage are usually of the base of the skull which often do not show on routine x-rays. Thus clinical examination and observation are of the greatest importance.

Fractures of the skull are only of importance when associated with damage to underlying structures. This damage is commonest when the base of the skull is involved. When the front of the skull is broken then

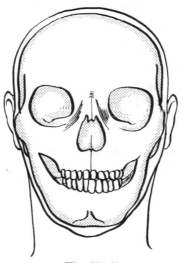

The Skull

often the cerebrospinal fluid escapes into the nose and the patient has watery nose bleeding. This can also allow germs from the nose to enter to the skull and so there is a risk of meningitis. If there is nerve damage then the patient loses his sense of smell while underlying brain damage results in loss of concentration and an instability of mood. If the middle part of the base of the skull is damaged then bleeding may occur from the ear, and the nerves supplying the muscles of the eye are liable to be damaged giving a squint and double vision or hearing may be lost. These latter injuries carry the risk of haemorrhage from the middle meningeal artery which is perhaps the most urgent of surgical emergencies. Fractures of the posterior part of the base of the skull are less common. They may cause injuries to the part of the brain concerned with vision or damage to the last four cranial nerves. The sign of fractures in this region is bruising round the back of the neck which only appears 24–48 hours after the injury.

After a head injury, whether or not a fracture is present, the patient may improve without further symptoms, he may remain in his present state or he may deteriorate. Deterioration is seen by the development of new signs or a deepening of the level of consciousness. Thus a patient who is conscious may become comatose or one who is unconscious may become more deeply unconscious. Therefore, as soon as possible the patient should be assessed to obtain a base line of his level of consciousness. Superficially one recognises that the patient is either conscious and well-orientated or unconscious but, in fact, unconsciousness has various levels. For instance, the patient while unable to speak can respond to painful stimuli or even if he cannot respond to painful stimuli his superficial and deep reflexes may be present. The degree of responsiveness to stimuli is one of the most useful indications in assessing whether or not a patient is improving after his head injury and because of this it is important not to give sedative drugs to these patients and upset the determination of the level of consciousness. Careful notes must be kept on the progress of the patient. Other factors which should be charted are half-hourly records of pulse rate, systolic blood pressure and respiration since there is often a tendency during compression of the brain due to bleeding for the pulse rate to show progressive slowing and the blood pressure to rise.

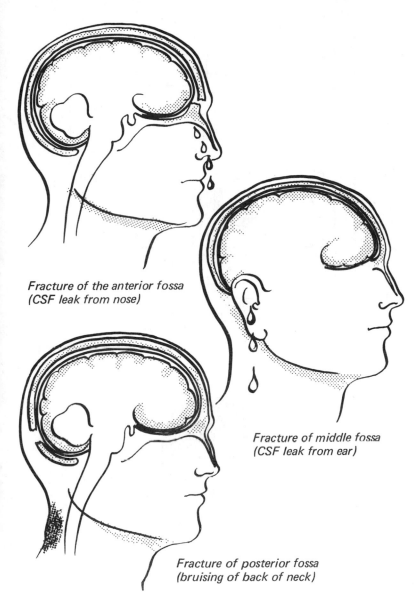

*Fracture of the anterior fossa
(CSF leak from nose)*

*Fracture of middle fossa
(CSF leak from ear)*

*Fracture of posterior fossa
(bruising of back of neck)*

147

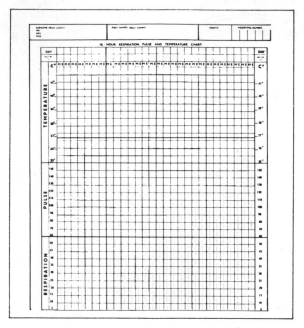

Another valuable sign which should be charted is the state of the pupils — whether they are dilated or contracted and whether they react to

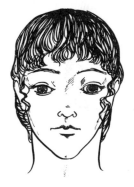

Fixed dilated pupil due to cerebral compression

light. If there is pressure on the brain then the pupil on the side of the blood clot is liable to become larger and to react more sluggishly to light than the pupil on the other side and it is most important to determine this early sign of impending danger. Other signs which can be listed to help in the care of the patient are the presence or absence of the reflexes and their character but these are better left to frequent medical examination by the doctor in charge of the patient. These patients may remain unconscious for a considerable length of time, varying from hours to weeks, months or even years and once it is established that little change is taking place in the patient the further maintenance largely becomes a matter of expert nursing.

The essentials in caring for any unconscious patient also apply to the patient with head injury. The only outcome of a head injury which calls for surgical intervention as an emergency is the development of intracranial bleeding which compresses the brain. This can be of two varieties. The most serious is the bleeding that occurs from a tear in the middle meningeal artery. This leads to rapid deterioration of the patient and death may occur within a matter of half an hour. Those attendant on the patient should always be on the lookout for signs of this development and this includes both the medical and the nursing staff. The signs are deepening unconsciousness, slowing of the pulse,

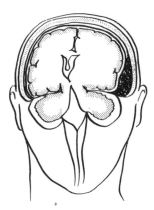

Extra-dural haematoma

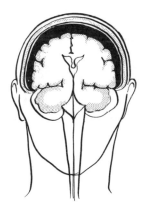

Sub-dural haematoma

rise of blood pressure and, most characteristically, dilation of the pupil on the same side as the bleeding with a sluggishness in reaction to light. However, the diagnosis should if possible be considered and made before the pupillary signs develop as they are due to serious compression of the brain and at this stage treatment may well have been too long delayed. The treatment is to open the skull and control the bleeding.

The other type of bleeding which can occur is into the space overlying the entire surface of the brain, the subdural space. Events here do not go so quickly and this may develop over a course of weeks or months. The bleeding is venous and is low pressure but leads to a deterioration in consciousness and mental state. The patient, in fact, has often regained consciousness and gone home from hospital when he becomes forgetful, confused and may indeed have symptoms mimicking psychiatric conditions. However, in hospital it may just lead to a slow diminution of the level of consciousness and the skull may have to be opened through numerous burrholes to establish whether or not a subdural haematoma is present and to extract the blood and wash out the space. This variety usually only occurs in older people in whom there is already some cerebral atrophy.

23
The Thyroid and Parathyroid Glands

Anatomy

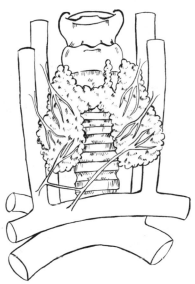

Anatomy of the thyroid gland.

The thyroid gland is situated in the front of the neck overlying the trachea. It consists of two lobes lying on either side of the trachea joined by a narrow strip called the isthmus. The gland is very vascular and each lobe is supplied by two large arteries, the superior and inferior thyroid vessels. Two nerves of importance are closely related to the gland on each side, the superior and recurrent laryngeal nerves which supply the muscles controlling the vocal cords in the larynx. Closely applied to the back of the gland are the four parathyroid glands, one in each corner.

The thyroid gland is an endocrine gland which produces a hormone, thyroxine. This hormone controls the metabolic rate of the body. Diseases of the gland result in either overproduction or underproduction of thyroxine, (i.e. hyperthyroidism or hypothyroidism). Enlargement

151

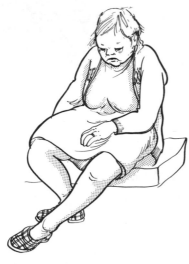

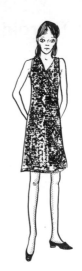

Myxoedema   *Thyrotoxicosis*

of the gland is called goitre, and may occur in either hyperthyroidism
or hypothyroidism or even when the function of the gland is normal
(simple goitre).

The treatment of hypothyroidism (myxoedema) is to give replacement thyroxine by mouth. The treatment of hyperthyroidism is also
medical by means of antithyroid drugs or radioactive iodine.
Antithyroid drugs are stopped before surgery and iodine given for a
week before operation.

There are three indications for surgery in thyroid diseases:—

    1. Failure of medical treatment in hyperthyroidism
    2. Pressure effects due to enlargement of the gland
    3. Thyroid tumour — these may be the simple adenoma or
       thyroid carcinoma.

The amount of gland removed depends on the extent of the disease.
Total thyroidectomy may be used in carcinoma, subtotal — removal of
90 — 95% of gland in thyrotoxicosis and lesser excisions for adenomas
and goitre.

The skin preparation involves the neck area and the axillae.

Post operatively the patient should be placed in a position with his neck supported until conscious.

Once conscious the patient should be sat up with the head and neck well supported to prevent strain on the suture line and the distressing feeling of losing his head. When the patient requires to move, turn, sit up or lie down, he should be assisted by nurse. By the second day he should be taught to support his own head and neck while moving but the nurse should always be on hand to give help when required. The drain in the incision is removed approximately one day after operation and the sutures or clips, four days after operation. After this, the patient may be encouraged to do gentle neck movements.

The patient is nursed in a well ventilated room with light coverings on the bed. His diet should initially be of high carbohydrate fluids, with a gradual introduction to soft diet as he will have difficulty in swallowing. Initially he may require intravenous fluids. The patient's throat will probably be sore and he may therefore be given a steam inhalation or throat lozenges to suck. Activity, if progress is satisfactory, should be encouraged within a few days of operation.

Thyroid surgery has certain complications peculiar to it and though relatively infrequent, if they do occur they are dangerous. First of these is the tendency to bleeding. The peculiar danger of haemorrhage in this situation is that the bleeding occurs into a closed space round the trachea and suffocation can quickly occur.

To observe for haemorrhage the patient should have a loose dressing over his wound and staining should be observed at the front and the back of the neck. The pulse, blood pressure and respirations should be recorded at 15 minute intervals. A choking sensation, difficulty in coughing or swallowing, a tight feeling in the neck, difficulty in breathing, cyanosis, a rise in the pulse rate and loss of consciousness will indicate that haemorrhage with obstruction to the air passages is taking place. This situation is very urgent and the nurse must loosen the dressing, immediately remove the middle stitches and open the wound to allow the escape of the blood. The nurse must not delay in doing this as delay means death to the patient. A tracheostomy set and stitch scissors or cutters must always be available.

The second complication is damage to the laryngeal nerves. If the superior nerves are damaged then an alteration in the voice occurs. Damage to one recurrent nerve results in a hoarse weak voice whereas bilateral damage results in loss of the voice and also inability to breathe properly as the paralysed vocal cords lie together and do not allow enough passage of air to the lungs. Thus bilateral nerve damage requires tracheostomy to allow adequate ventilation.

The third complication is removal of or damage to, the parathyroid glands. The patient feels tingling in the hands and feet, and spasm of the fingers, hands, toes and feet may occur (carpo-pedal spasm). The

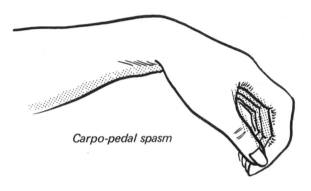

Carpo-pedal spasm

treatment is to administer calcium, and this may be given intravenously for rapid action and continued by mouth.

The last complication is fortunately becoming very rare and is called a thyroid crisis. This results from release of a massive amount of thyroxine into the blood during the operation. The patient literally burns himself up — the temperature soars, the heart rate rises to 140 − 200 beats per minute, the patient is flushed, sweating, anxious, and the slightest stimulation even by noise may produce a convulsion. Heart failure soon occurs if control is not quickly achieved. The patient is sedated to anaesthetic levels, intravenous cortisone, propanalol, and iodine are administered and nursing carried out in a quiet dark room with minimal disturbance until the crisis passes. Even with adequate treatment death not infrequently occurs. The chance of this complication occurring is very much less if the patient has normal thyroid function at the time of operation and so a careful pre-operative medical regime with antithyroid drugs and iodine is important.

The parathyroid glands also produce a hormone (parathormone) which controls the levels of calcium and phosphorus in the body. If the glands are overactive due to hyperplasie or more commonly to a tumour (parathyroid adenoma) then hyperparathyroidism occurs. This results in the formation of bone cysts (osteitis fibrosa cystica) and renal calculi amongst other rarer manifestations. The treatment is excision of the parathyroid tumour. This may be extremely difficult to find as the glands are very small and may be anywhere in the neck or even in the chest.

24
The Oesophagus

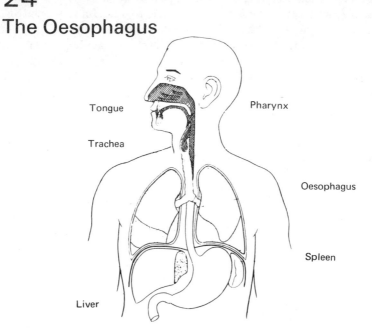

The oesophagus (or gullet) is a muscular tube which conveys the swallowed food or fluids to the stomach. It starts behind the larynx in the neck and runs through the chest behind the trachea, great vessels, and heart to enter the abdomen through the left diaphragm.

Diseases of the oesophagus or gullet, which involve the surgeon, are usually inflammation (oesophagitis) or tumour (carcinoma) of the oesophagus. In both these conditions the patient comes to the surgeon because of difficulty in swallowing (dysphagia). This usually starts with difficulty in swallowing foods such as meat, bread and then becomes progressively worse until only semi-solids can be taken. Finally only fluids can be swallowed. Meanwhile the patient, unable to get adequate nutrition loses weight, becomes thin and emaciated and because of the lack of intake of meat lacks iron and becomes anaemic. The symptoms of the two conditions are thus the same and differentiation depends on investigation. The investigations carried out are to x-ray the oesophagus while the patient swallows a mouthful of radio-opaque material, barium sulphate. In the case of oesophagitis, there is often a long narrow stricture at the lower end of the oesophagus due to burning of the oesophagus by acid coming up from the stomach. The stricture is smooth and regular. On the other hand, cancer of the oesophagus produces a stricture also but this is long and irregular and the appearances tend to be typical. If, however, there is any doubt the diagnosis can be confirmed

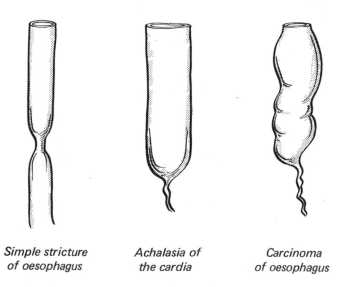

Simple stricture
of oesophagus

Achalasia of
the cardia

Carcinoma
of oesophagus

by oesophagoscopy. This involves the passage under general anaesthesia of a rigid tube down the oesophagus when the lesion can be seen under direct vision and a biopsy taken of any suspicious area.

Oesophagitis

Oesophagitis invariably results from the acid regurgitating from the stomach into the lower end of the gullet producing inflammation, which in turn causes fibrosis and results in the formation of a stricture. This is often associated with duodenal ulcer, and the commonest cause is a protrusion of the stomach through the diaphragm into the chest known as a Hiatus Hernia. In the early stages of the condition, it is often possible to relieve the stricture by the passage of gum elastic

157

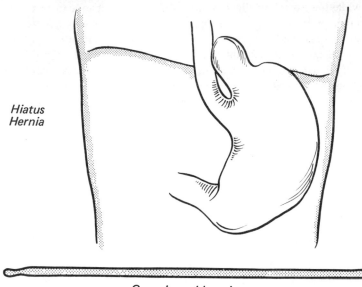

Hiatus Hernia

Oesophageal bougie

bougies to stretch the oesophagus up to a size which will allow the swallowing of normal food although this has often to be accompanied by treatment aimed at reducing the acidity of the stomach. If a hiatus hernia is present then it of course requires correction. Surgically this is done by reducing the stomach back into the abdominal cavity and repairing the gap in the diaphragm through which it has protruded. This is often accompanied by a vagotomy to reduce the acid in the stomach and some form of drainage operation such as pyloroplasty or gastro-enterostomy to prevent stasis in the stomach resulting from the vagotomy (see surgery of the stomach). If the stricture is too rigid to allow it to be stretched then excision of the stricture may be required with rejoining (anastomosis) of the oesophagus back onto the stomach.

Cancer of the Oesophagus

Cancer can occur anywhere in the oesophagus and generally speaking we divide it into three groups. That occuring in the upper third, that occuring in the middle third and that occuring in the lower third. Generally speaking, cancer of the upper two thirds of the

158

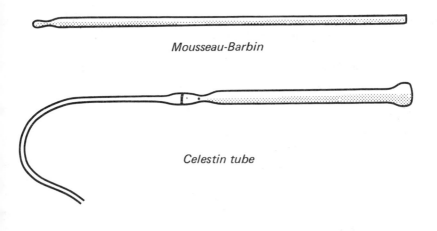

Mousseau-Barbin

Celestin tube

oesophagus is better dealt with by radiotherapy but in the lower third of
the oesophagus, surgery is the usual treatment and consists of excising
the lower third of the oesophagus and the upper end of the stomach and
re-anastomosing the oesophagus to the stomach. If there is not enough
tissue to allow the oesophagus to be anastomosed to the stomach then
some other part of the bowel is interposed to allow continuity to be
re-established. After operations on the oesophagus nothing must be
swallowed for 4 – 5 days. If the tumour is inoperable then useful
palliation can be achieved by the passage of a plastic tube through the
tumour. The two tubes in common use are known as a Mousseau-
Barbin and a Celestin tube. Both of these tubes have funnels at the
upper end and wide lumens and they are passed through the tumour so
that the funnel is above it and the wide lower end opens into the
stomach and this allows the passage of food stuffs and abolishes the
symptom of dysphagia. This is usefully combined with radiotherapy.
The patient will be allowed sips of water on return from theatre but
after twelve hours will have a fluid diet introduced, and should soon

cope with a semi-solid diet. To keep his tube clean and clear he should be instructed to have plain water with his meals and to take a fizzy drink after it to dislodge any food particles. All operations on the oesophagus involve an incision into the chest and the operation is carried out through one or other pleural cavity. The lung being collapsed and retracted out of the way. The operation is therefore a serious one. Before surgery the patient's general condition may be improved by giving a varied, well balanced diet. A record of fluid intake and output, weight recording and measures to prevent the formation of pressure sores must be employed as the patient will often be malnourished on admission. Regurgitation of foodstuffs may occur, so regular mouthwashes are given to keep the mouth fresh. Intravenous feeding, gastric suction, oxygen therapy and regular breathing exercises are important aspects of post-operative care. A water seal chest drain will be used in the post-operative phase. The sutures may be removed after ten to fourteen days. The main complication of operations on the oesophagus is a leak from the anastomosis. The Oesophagus has a deficient weak outer muscular coat and heals badly. If a leak occurs then infection involves the mediastinum and leads to a very severe infection there which often results in the death of the patient.

25
Stomach and Duodenum

Structure and Function

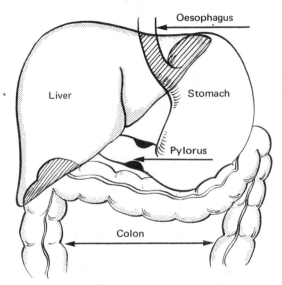

Relations of the stomach and duodenum

The stomach is in the upper abdomen and receives the ingested food from the oesophagus at its upper end where there is normally a sphincteric action to prevent regurgitation of acid into the oesophagus, this sphincter is called the cardia. The exit from the stomach into the duodenum is also guarded by a sphincter called the pylorus. The function of the stomach is to act as a reservoir for the ingested food, to mix it, acidify it and kill its bacterial content. In the stomach digestion of carbohydrates continues, the digestion of protein commences and some simple substances such as alcohol and some drugs are absorbed. When the contents are passed on to the duodenum they are neuturalised by alkaline secretions and emulsified by mixing with bile. The bile is accompanied at its entrance to the duodenum at the ampulla of Vater by the secretions of the pancreas. This contains enzymes for the digestion

of fat, carbohydrates and the further breakdown of proteins. The
duodenal contents then pass into the small bowel where digestion
continues and absorption commences.

The nerve supply of the stomach is from the vagus nerves which run
down the front and back of the oesophagus. They control the acid
output and movements of the stomach.

Diseases of Stomach and Duodenum

The diseases of stomach and duodenum which require surgery are in
the main peptic ulceration and cancer. Peptic ulcers are found in both
stomach and duodenum, but cancer affects the stomach only. The
operations performed are those of gastrectomy, either   partial or total,
and vagotomy with drainage (pyloroplasty or gastrojejunostomy).
— see appendix.

Investigation

Special investigation of diseases of stomach and duodenum involve
the swallowing of a radio-opaque medium to outline the bowel followed
by x-ray screening (a barium meal), the passage of an instrument via the
mouth and oesophagus under local anaesthesia to allow inspection of the
lining of the stomach (gastroscopy or fibroscopy) and the giving of
substances such as histamine or pentagastrin to produce the maximum
amount of acid possible and to aspirate at intervals over a period of
time for chemical examination (a test meal). In patients who have had
a vagotomy a variety of test meal is performed where the stimulus is an
intravenous injection of insulin. This allows one to decide
whether denervation of the stomach is complete.

Peptic Ulcer

The cause of peptic ulcer is unknown. It has been ascribed to
stress, to diet, to excesses of alcohol or smoking, and it is likely that all
of these may be involved. Ulcers in the stomach may be acute or
chronic and may give rise to cancer or cancer may start as an ulcer. It
is therefore important that an ulcer which does not show signs of
healing with medical treatment should be examined by the pathologist
without undue delay. If a gastric ulcer does not show signs of healing in
six weeks on a full medical regime, then a surgical opinion is sought.

On the other hand duodenal ulcer never gives rise to cancer and the treatment is primarily medical. Most ulcers will heal with a regime of diet, antacids and drugs which block the vagus nerve, and surgery is only required for those which do not heal, or those which develop complications. It should be noted that medical treatment cannot be considered successful unless the patient can lead a normal life with an unrestricted diet. A lifetime of bland diet and pills constitutes a gastric cripple rather than a successfully treated ulcer patient.

The indications for surgery in peptic ulcer are therefore —

    a Failure of medical treatment
    b Haematemesis and/or melaena
    c Perforation
    d Pyloric stenosis

Failure of Medical Treatment

In gastric ulcer this means failure to improve symptomatically or absence of healing on barium meal or gastroscopy in six to twelve weeks.

In duodenal ulcer, which characteristically pursues a long chronic course with remissions and relapses, a period of up to two years on a medical regime should be followed before surgery is considered.

Haematemesis

This means the vomiting of blood, either fresh or "coffee grounds", while melaena means the passage of altered blood per rectum. There are many causes for these complaints, but bleeding from a peptic ulcer is by far the commonest. The bleeding occurs when the ulcer erodes the wall of a blood vessel in its base. This may happen spontaneously or be precipitated by the ingestion of drugs such as aspirin or alcohol. The bleeding may be catastrophic and fatal if a large vessel is eroded, or a slow continuous ooze leading to anaemia. The former more commonly gives rise to haematemesis and the latter to melaena. The patient who vomits blood shows all the signs of shock. He is cold, clammy, sweating, with ashen pallor and a rapid pulse and low blood pressure. He will give a history of dyspepsia or salicylate ingestion. The initial treatment is medical. He should be put to bed, sedated with morphia and reassured. The stomach is emptied with a nasogastric tube and thereafter hourly aspiration carried out to check if bleeding is still present. This with advantage can be combined with the instillation of ice cold water at each aspiration. The blood pressure and pulse are checked half-hourly and the haemoglobin and packed cell volume are checked daily. Blood transfusion is given to replace blood loss and this is particularly important if surgery is being considered. The patient is closely observed. If bleeding continues in spite of the above regime, then surgery is indicated. It is also usually required in patients over the age of 60 years, who stand blood loss badly. Mostly, in haematemesis, the bleeding will stop spontaneously and the patient nursed back to health. A decision must then be made whether to continue medical treatment or carry out elective surgery. If the patient has had a previous haematemesis, or perforation, or is over 65 years, then surgery is necessary, but in the younger patient where this is the first complication, or where a medical regime has not been adequately tried, then medical treatment is indicated. Between these extremes each case must be judged on its merits. Perhaps the greatest advance in the treatment of haematemesis in recent years has been the practice of calling for a surgical opinion when the patient is first admitted. The patient's progress can then be reviewed by physician and surgeon together and the appropriate course of action at each stage be jointly decided.

If surgery becomes necessary the choice of operation is dictated by the findings at laparotomy.

Perforation

This complication occurs during acute ulceration and may be the first indication the patient has that all is not well in his stomach. The ulcer erodes the wall of the stomach or duodenum and allows the infective acid contents to spill into the peritoneal cavity giving rise to a severe peritonitis. Clinically the presentation is dramatic, the patient is suddenly seized with severe abdominal pain and becomes shocked and collapsed. The pain is so severe he lies still, afraid to move, his face pale and drawn and covered with cold sweat. The pulse is rapid and thready, the blood pressure low and the abdomen is held rigidly like a board. A straight x-ray of abdomen at this time will often show free gas in the peritoneal cavity, or a gastrografin examination may show spillage of dye from the ulcer — but these seldom do more than confirm the obvious clinical picture. There is no place for medical treatment in perforation, the mortality rises alarmingly after 12 hours and operation should not be unduly delayed.

The patient is admitted and given relief from pain by means of an injection of morphia or papaveretum. A nasogastric tube is passed and suction commenced to empty the stomach and prevent further soiling of the peritoneum. An intravenous infusion is commenced and shock corrected if necessary by means of macrodex. Operation should be performed as soon as possible. The standard operative treatment is to clean the peritoneal cavity of contamination by sucking out the leaked gastric contents and to repair the perforation by simple suturing of the hole. Many patients never require further surgery. Apart from the complications which may occur after any abdominal surgery, perforation may lead to the development of a subphrenic abscess. This is an abscess which forms between the diaphragm and the liver on the right side or between diaphragm, stomach and spleen on the left. It is due to the spilt gastric contents setting up infection in these sites. It leads to immobility of the diaphragm with collapse of the overlying lung and perhaps pneumonia. The patient becomes extremely ill and toxic with a high swinging temperature and rapid weight loss. Antibiotics alone are of little value and treatment consists of localisation and drainage of the abscess.

Pyloric stenosis

This condition complicates duodenal ulcer and occurs when the ulcer heals. The gross scarring and fibrosis which result lead to narrowing of the pylorus. The wall of the stomach thickens to force the contents through the narrowing channel and becomes enlarged. As the obstruction becomes complete the stomach cannot empty and becomes dilated until it is a large immobile bag containing the decomposing remnants of many meals. The patient gives a history of past indigestion which has changed its character. The pain has gone to be replaced by vomiting, at first intermittent but eventually and characteristically by the projectile vomiting of large volumes of foul gastric contents in which remnants of meals eaten many hours, or indeed days before are still recognisable. Accompanying this is weight loss, malnutrition and severe electrolyte imbalance due to the continuous loss of acid from the stomach. In mild cases a barium meal will show a vast dilated stomach in which the barium lies as a pool. In severe cases the diagnosis is obvious clinically and further investigation unnecessary. The treatment of pyloric stenosis is surgery. But first the stomach must be cleared by lavage via a gastric tube and the electrolyte upset restored to normal by an intravenous infusion of saline. When the patient's dehydration, and electrolyte deficiency have been corrected, then operation to relieve the obstruction is performed. This is usually a gastrojejunostomy, vagotomy being unnecessary as the ulcer has healed.

A similar condition can occur in newborn infants due to a thickened pyloric sphincter which fails to relax. This is called hypertrophic pyloric stenosis, and is relieved by simply dividing the pyloric sphincter without opening the lumen of the bowel (pyloromyotomy or Rammstedt operation).

Carcinoma of stomach

Cancer of the stomach may arise in a pre-existing ulcer, but most often occurs in a previously healthy stomach. It is insidious and initially it produces little in the way of symptoms, mild dyspepsia, a distaste for food especially meat, weight loss and lack of energy. The pain when it occurs is not relieved by alkalis as in ulcer. Vomiting occurs and may contain blood. Blood loss occurs steadily in the stools giving rise to anaemia. The downhill course is rapid and most patients are beyond the stage of cure when first seen. The tumour may be felt, may be demonstrated by barium meal or fibroscopy. A test meal shows absence of free hydrochloric acid in the stomach. The outlook in this disease is poor, only 10% of patients being alive 5 years after treatment. Curative treatment is by subtotal or total gastrectomy, along with the spleen and neighbouring lymphatic glands. This carries a high mortality and is less often performed. In most cases palliative surgery is all that is feasible. Wherever possible this should be a partial gastrectomy to remove the tumour, but where this is impossible a gastro-enterostomy may be performed for growths low in the stomach or for growths near the oesophagus a plastic tube may be threaded through the tumour to allow the patient to swallow (Souttars, Mousseau-Barbin tube). In many cases with liver secondaries, peritoneal spread or ascites (fluid filling the abdominal cavity) nothing at all can be done and the abdomen is closed. Radiotherapy and cytotoxic drugs have little to offer in the treatment of carcinoma of stomach.

When operation is necessary for ulcer then either a partial

gastrectomy or vagotomy with a drainage operation is performed. Each has its drawbacks.

1. Partial gastrectomy reduces the volume of the stomach so that meals must be small in amount and taken frequently if undernourishment is not to result. It also removes the intrinsic factor necessary for the absorption of vitamins essential in blood formation and so a long term result is anaemia rather like. pernicious anaemia.

2. The main problem accompanying vagotomy is the risk of episodic urgent diarrhoea, the stools being pale in colour. This may affect 10 – 20% of patients having a vagotomy. Nevertheless, 95% of patients are delighted with the results of gastric surgery, and can once again enjoy and relish their food.

Nursing Care Following Gastric or Duodenal Surgery

Pre-operative Care

If the operation is an elective one, nurse may help to improve the patient's nutritional status by giving frequent small nourishing meals and fluids or the patient may require artificial feeding. Whether the operation is an emergency one or not the patient may very well have a transfusion or commence intravenous fluids prior to operation.

It is important that the patient's mouth is clean and free from sepsis. If the patient's admission is an emergency one, routine cleaning of the patient's mouth should be carried out, however, if the patient is having an elective operation dental care should be given if possible prior to admission and oral hygiene attended to frequently after admission. As smoking and alcohol probably irritate the stomach lining the patient should not indulge in either. Smoking also predisposes to chest infections and since the patient's operation will interfere with the abdominal muscles this will restrict his breathing to a certain extent. The stomach lies directly beneath the diaphragm so breathing postoperatively may be painful. Breathing exercises should therefore be taught and commenced before going to theatre and the patient will also be instructed on how to move around the bed and perform leg exercises. This will help to prevent chest complications and venous complications post-operatively.

Vomiting may be a feature of the disease pre-operatively so careful attention to observation of the time, amount, the character, the type and the relation of the vomiting to food or drugs given, should be noted. Any pain which the patient may complain of should be reported, with an indication of the site, the character and the duration.

It will depend on the type of operation being performed and whether it is an emergency operation or not whether bowel preparation will be given. If, particularly in the case of elective surgery, bowel care is required, a suppository to be given on the evening prior to operation may be ordered by doctor. The pubic, abdominal and lower chest regions should be shaved and cleaned and special attention paid to the cleanliness of the umbilicus.

The patient's stomach will be emptied by aspiration after passage of a Levine's tube. If, however, the patient is suffering from a pyloric stenosis a gastric lavage will be required prior to surgery.

Many of these patients will have had a chest x-ray or a series of barium films and these should accompany the patient to theatre. Emergency treatment of particular conditions has already been mentioned.

Post-Operative Care

All routine post operative care would be required by this patient. The pulse and blood pressure must be recorded half-hourly initially on the patient's return from theatre and routine care given to the transfusion or intravenous infusion of fluids.

The patient may have continuous or intermittent gastric suction and nurse must remember never to let the suction rise above 5 centimetres of mercury and always to note carefully the amount of suction required in any particular hour. The aspiration should be observed carefully and any blood or bile which is present should be reported. Alternatively the nasogastric tube may be left to drain freely into a drainage bag. The naso-gastric tube is left in position until doctor is satisfied that the alimentary tract is again functioning reasonably satisfactorily and it is usually removed after 24 to 48 hours post operatively. The intravenous fluids are continued for 1 to 3 days but after perhaps about 8 to 12 hours the patient may be allowed 30 millilitres of water orally. An explanation must be given to the patient about the importance of taking only the amount of fluids which he is allowed and if his relatives are also told of this their co-operation can also be gained. The patient will slowly graduate to larger quantities of water, water and milk mixture, non irritating fluids, on to a semi-solid diet and by the end of about a week he is able to take a light, easily digested diet.

The patient's bowels generally move within 4 days of operation but if this does not occur doctor may order a suppository.

The patient must be maintained on a fluid balance chart until normal feeding is resumed and careful note should be made of the amount, the character and any abnormalities in the gastric aspirate or in the urine.

The patient is encouraged to move after operation and is often allowed up to sit on the first or the second day for a short time. He should be encouraged to move in his bed and while confined to it special care must be taken of the skin and of the patient's general hygiene. After about seven days the patient is generally able to move around on his own.

The patient is on restricted fluids and gastric suction in the immediate post-operative phase and is therefore losing fluid, and is not having any washing through his mouth. His oral hygiene must therefore be given particular attention by the nurse until the patient is having an adequate intake and can care for it himself.

Immediately after operation routine observations of the wound would be carried out. The dressing is generally left untouched for about ten days and the sutures then removed. If the patient has a small wound drain in position this would be left for three days.

The patient is generally allowed home, if his condition is satisfactory, at the end of two to three weeks and this spell in hospital should be followed by convalescence. Return to work is usually not advised until after 4 to 6 weeks. The patient must be given a date for return for follow up care and this is particularly important if he has a malignancy.

On discharge from hospital the patient is often advised to take frequent small easily digested meals and gradually accustom himself to a fairly normal routine of eating. If, however, the patient has had a major part of his stomach removed he may require to take small frequent meals for the rest of his life.

26
The Small Bowel and Appendix

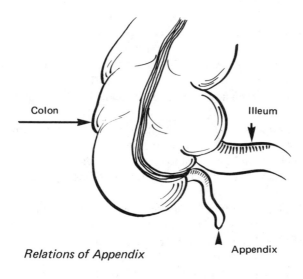

Colon

Illeum

Appendix

Relations of Appendix

The small bowel is remarkably free from disease. Apart from infections such as gastroenteritis, typhoid, and tuberculosis which do not involve the surgeon, tumours are uncommon and usually present as obstructions which require laparotomy.

A disease which also causes small bowel obstruction is regional ileitis or Crohn's disease. This is an inflammation of the bowel of unknown cause which affects the bowel here and there and heals by fibrosis leading to obstruction. The treatment is to excise the affected parts. Unfortunately the condition usually recurs and these patients require repeated excisions over the years.

Appendicitis can conveniently be considered at this point. The appendix hangs from the tip of the caecum just below the junction of ileum and caecum and is about 8 cms. long. It is a little cul de sac of the alimentary tract and very prone to infection. Appendicitis occurs at any age but is uncommon at the extremes of life. The patient develops vague central abdominal pain, and is often sick. The pain then becomes constant and moves down to become localised in the right lower abdomen. It may be associated with diarrhoea and frequency of micturition if the appendix lies low in the pelvis. The temperature is slightly raised as is the pulse. On examination there is marked tenderness over the appendix. The treatment is removal of the appendix. If the infection is severe or treatment delayed the appendix may rupture to give rise to generalised peritonitis. This is a severe and possibly fatal complication and requires appendicectomy and drainage of the peritoneal cavity in addition to antibiotics and general supportive measures. If the development of the disease is slower then an abscess may form round the appendix. This is a contra indication to immediate surgery. The patient is treated conservatively with antibiotics and usually the condition settles in seven to ten days. The appendicectomy is then carried out in three months time. During the course of this conservative treatment however, any sign of deterioration such as a rising temperature or increase in the size of the abscess is an indication for immediate surgery. This treatment must always therefore be carried out in hospital where a theatre can always be available at short notice.

In acute appendicitis or indeed any intra-abdominal sepsis, abscesses may form in the peritoneal cavity. The common sites are under the diaphragm (subphrenic abscess) or in the pelvis (pelvic abscess). The patient fails to improve and develops a high swinging temperature. Those under the diaphragm are associated with dyspnoea and collapse of the lung cases while pelvic abscess is associated with diarrhoea. The treatment is incision and drainage. A pelvic abscess is opened through the rectum or vagina. A subphrenic abscess through the most appropriate site depending whether it is left or right, anterior or posterior.

Obstruction

Obstruction is one of the common surgical emergencies usually occuring in patients in the second half of life although there are varieties of obstructions which are congenital and affect the new born. Obstruction means that the lumen of the bowel is occluded and the onward passage of the contents is halted. The bowel above the obstruction distends and fills up with the intestinal secretions until eventually the patient starts vomiting. While this is happening the bowel below the obstruction empties itself and then ceases to function. Even before the patient starts vomiting, the bowel is distending with intestinal juices and this means that there is a nett loss of salt and water to the body.

The cause of the obstruction to the bowel may be something in the lumen of the bowel itself, such as a swallowed foreign body, or a mass of indigested foodstuffs, or it may be arising in the wall of the bowel — such as a tumour, prolapsing into the lumen, or a tumour producing a stricture. Or, most commonly of all, the obstruction may arise from something external to the bowel producing the lesion by pressure, such as a band or adhesion or the effect of a neck of a hernia obstructing the bowel. Regardless of the cause, the symptoms are the same and the only differentiation in symptoms occur in whether the obstruction is high in the small bowel or low in the large bowel. In high small bowel obstruction vomiting occurs early and the patient quickly becomes collapsed, dehydrated and in water and salt imbalance. On the other hand, if the obstruction is in the colon the abdomen distends, the patient is constipated with no passage of flatus and vomiting occurs relatively late. In large bowel obstructions the distension may be confined to the large bowel since the valve between the ileum and the caecum may prevent pressure being transmitted back to the small bowel. When this is the case the large bowel may rupture, leading to a very fatal type of peritonitis. If the valve is incompetent the pressure can be transmitted back to the small bowel and the patient shows all the signs of small bowel obstruction. The diagnosis is usually obvious from the patient's abdominal distension, history of severe vomiting and absolute constipation. Confirmatory evidence can be gained by a straight x-ray of the abdomen taken in the upright position, when loops of bowel can be seen containing fluids and gas with a straight line junction between the two — these are known as fluid levels. The treatment of intestinal obstruction is laparotomy and the relief of the obstruction. This may involve the simple division of a band, the repair of a hernia or may involve excision of a portion of bowel. In some instances the obstructing agent cannot easily be removed, in which case part of the dilated bowel above the obstruction is anastomosed to the collapsed bowel beyond the obstruction, effecting a bypass. When a bypass has been done it is some-times feasible to carry out a second operation subsequently to remove the affected portion of bowel. If the lesion is a tumour of the large bowel then often the most effective way of relieving the obstruction is to bring the large bowel above the obstruction to the surface of the skin and allow the intestinal contents to discharge there; this is known as a colostomy and in this instance is usually made in the form of a loop, so that when it is opened there are two openings visible on the surface of the skin — the proximal one discharging faeces and the distal one leading down to the area of the obstruction. When the patient is obstructed the colostomy requires to be opened as soon as possible and, to avoid soiling the wound with masses of liquid faeces, a tube is often inserted into the colon and led to a bag at the bedside, so that the gas and faecal material can be led away from the recent wound; this is known as a Paul's tube. In less acute cases the colostomy can be left unopened for three to four days until the wound has had a chance to seal off the bowel; it is then opened with diathermy and this does not require an anaesthetic and can be done in the ward or sideroom of theatre. If the blood supply to the bowel is occluded, as happens in hernias, then the bowel becomes gangrenous and strangulation is said to have occured. The treatment is then to relieve the obstruction and resect the gangrenous bowel.

Other special types of obstruction which can also result in strangulation are:

    a Volvulus — Where a loop of bowel becomes twisted on itself.

    b Intussusception — Where a portion of bowel becomes drawn into a neighbouring portion of bowel as if it were bowel contents.

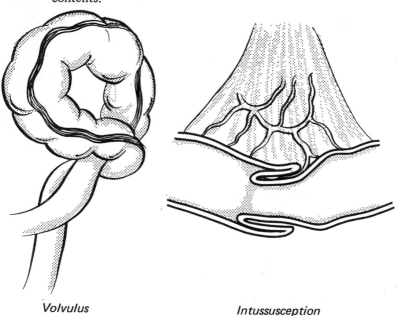

Volvulus   *Intussusception*

27
The Colon

Anatomy and Physiology

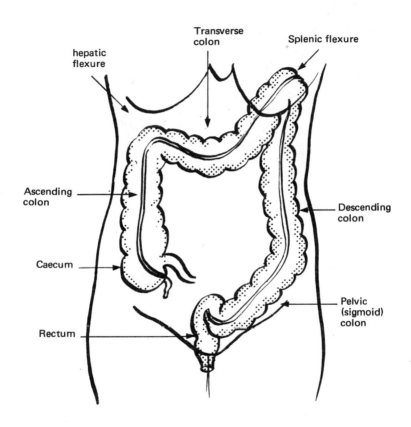

The colon starts in the right iliac fossa where it is called the caecum. It is joined here by the terminal ileum whose entrance is in the form of a valve which normally only allows forward transit of the contents. Attached to the tip of the caecum is the appendix. The colon runs up the right posterior abdominal wall to the liver and then turns medially and downwards at the hepatic flexure to become the transverse colon. This part of the colon runs across the abdomen to the splenic flexure when it again runs downwards along the left posterior wall of the abdomen to the left iliac fossa where it swings out in a curve known as the pelvic colon to join the upper end of the rectum at the pelvic floor. The right and left colon are firmly fixed to the posterior abdominal wall and only have peritoneum on their front whereas the transverse and pelvic colon are suspended from the posterior abdominal wall by a fold of peritoneum which surrounds them and so are intra abdominal and mobile. The wall of the colon is deficient in its muscular layers, the outer longitudinal inside being represented by three bands known as taeniae. The blood supply of the colon as far as the splenic flexure is from the superior mesenteric artery which also supplies the small bowel. The rest of the colon is supplied from the inferior mesenteric artery which also supplies the rectum. The lymph drainage from the colon follows the blood vessels back to the aorta.

Diseases of the Colon

There is a wide spectrum of colonic disease ranging from the infective diarrhoeas and dysenteries to the non-specific conditions such as ulcerative colitis and Crohn's disease and to the tumours of bowel. All diseases of the colon, however, have certain features in common. The colon reacts to irritation, whether it be by infection or by tumour, by producing an outflow of mucus and diarrhoea. Superadded on this, however, may be constipation if the condition of the colon occludes the lumen. Most of the conditions also tend to cause bleeding, either the loss of fresh red blood per rectum, or the passage of altered blood (melaena).

The diseases which principally concern the surgeon are — in the non-specific group, Crohn's disease, ulcerative colitis, diverticulitis, and in the tumours, carcinoma of colon and rectum.

Ulcerative Colitis

This well known condition affects mainly young adults, though there is a second peak of occurence in the fifties. It is characterised by intractable diarrhoea frequently containing blood and mucus. The whole colon is usually involved and is extensively ulcerated and lined by granulation tissue. This leads to the passage of large amounts of mucus and blood per rectum. The number of stools may be $10 - 20$ a day and many of them consists only of mucus and blood. The patient rapidly becomes toxic, and emaciated, the weight loss may be extremely gross and the patient may weigh only $4 - 5$ stones in the severest form of the disease. In some varieties of the disease the course is rapid and acute, but more commonly it runs a slow, intermittent course with bouts of acute exacerbations and periods of quiescence. The prime treatment of the disease is medical with the use of sulphonamides, such as sulphasalazine, and steroids, such as cortisone, either given systemically or by means of enemata. This specific treatment is coupled with supportive treatment in the way of a high protein diet and symptomatic treatment of the diarrhoea by simple medicaments, such as kaolin, chalk and opium, or syrup of codeine phosphate. Vitamins require to be supplied since there is a loss of normal bacterial flora of the bowel producing vitamins and lack of absorption of these.

The surgeon is called in in the acute fulminating disease where the course may not be altered by medical treatment. His services are also required in the very chronic form of the disease where the patient eventually has a colon which is rigid and fibrosed due to healing of the ulceration and resembles a hose-pipe. This also leads to intractable diarrhoea. More significant, perhaps, is the fact that the patient with chronic ulcerative colitis is much more prone to develop cancer of the bowel than the normal subject. Unfortunately the only surgical way of curing the condition is by means of a total colectomy and proctectomy. This means that the bowel ends at the terminal ileum which must then be brought out on to the surface of the body as an artificial anus, called an ileostomy. This involves many difficulties which will be discussed later.

Crohn's Disease

Crohn's disease in the large bowel tends to lead to stricture formation and obstruction and the symptoms are those of obstruction of the large bowel, the diagnosis being made by means of an x-ray (barium enema) showing a stricture of bowel, or more commonly at Laparotomy for obstruction. The treatment is resection of the affected colon.

Diverticular Disease of the Colon

This is an extremely common disease, usually commencing in the middle years of life and becoming progressively more common until it affects perhaps 40 per cent of the population in the late sixties. Basically it is caused by lack of peristalsis and localised spasm resulting in areas of high pressure in the bowel which push out little pouches of mucosa between the circular muscle fibres. These diverticulae give the characteristic appearance on x-ray of little pockets of barium lying outwith the lumen of the bowel. The disease in many cases is asymptomatic, but most commonly the patient is constipated and this constipation leads to the retention of faeces in the little diverticulae which set up an inflammatory response. This results in transient diarrhoea. The spasm of the colon is also associated with colicky pain most commonly in the left iliac fossa. If the inflammation in the diverticulum progresses a small abscess may be formed resulting in the condition of pericolic abscess. This leads to severe diarrhoea and symptomatic upset with a high swinging fever, raised pulse rate and pain over the affected colon. The formation of a pericolic abscess leads to adhesion of the surrounding structures to the outer wall of the abscess, commonly small bowel and bladder. The abscess may rupture externally, which is uncommon, or may be drained surgically. Frequently the abscess bursts into the surrounding loops of small bowel or bladder to give rise to one of the worst complications of this disease − a fistula, either to small bowel leading to intractable diarrhoea, or to bladder leading to a very severe form of cystitis, pyelitis and the passage of air in the urine, known as pneumaturia.

Inflammation in the diverticulae may also cause erosion of the neighbouring blood vessels, leading characteristically to a very large sudden haemorrhage from the bowel which usually stops spontaneously without surgical intervention. On the other hand, in the absence of this complication there is commonly a small continuous blood loss, leading

178

to a chronic type of iron deficiency anaemia.

The treatment of diverticular disease, in the absence of complications, is medical. Treatment is directed towards keeping the bowel distended and full and preventing the faeces becoming inspissated and hard. To this end the patient is given a high residue diet containing bran products and the use of colloidal aperients such as Isogel and Celevac to increase the bulk of the faeces and keep them soft. Painful spasms of the bowel that occur can be treated by the drugs preventing spasm such as propantheline or dicyclomine, while for the acute attacks of inflammation broad spectrum antibiotics such as ampicillin or tetracycline are indicated. The former treatment with non-absorbable sulphonamides is now believed to be of little value. If the disease is localised to one segment of the bowel, and this is commonly the sigmoid colon, then the results of the surgery in the first instance are now good and resection of the affected segment is perhaps the treatment of choice. Commonly, however, the disease affects a large area of the bowel and resection is not feasible. In these cases surgery is only indicated for the complications, either pericolic abscess or fistula formation.

Occasionally, healing of inflammatory areas of the bowel can be accompanied by stricture formation and so the patient with diverticular disease can also present as a large bowel obstruction and in these cases it is often extremely difficult, both on barium enema and indeed at laparotomy to decide whether the condition is simple or malignant.

The treatment of fistulas and inflammation in the colon commonly requires a staged operation. In the first instance the faecal stream is diverted by means of a transverse colostomy to allow the bowel to become quiescent and the inflammation to subside. Some weeks later, when the patient's condition has improved, then a resection of the diseased part of the bowel is carried out, the fistula is repaired, and then the colostomy is closed to allow the faeces to pass by the natural route.

Carcinoma

Carcinoma of the large bowel is a common condition. It can affect any part of the bowel, the commonest site being perhaps the pelvic colon, followed in order of frequency by caecum and ascending colon and then by the left colon. There are two distinct kinds of carcinoma which occur. In the right half of the colon the carcinoma tends to be of the large fungating variety and this produces bleeding and general ill-health, but little in the way of dramatic signs of pain or obstruction. These patients are often admitted under the care of the physicians for investigation for iron deficiency anaemia and the cause is found to be a tumour in the right half of the colon. The treatment for tumours of the right colon is right hemi-colectomy. On the other hand, on the left half of the colon the tumour which most commonly occurs is a carcinoma which grows slowly round the bowel and narrows it down until it completely occludes the lumen. These tumours produce alternating constipation and diarrhoea and also occasional blood loss. They progress steadily towards complete obstruction and many present as emergencies on surgical receiving days as large bowel obstructions. Both of these types of tumour are shown on barium enema and this is the main means of diagnosis. Tumours of the left half of the colon are treated by left hemi-colectomy. For tumours in the pelvic colon and transverse colon, it is not necessary to resect the whole half colon, but only to remove the colon on either side of the tumour — partial colectomy.

The diagnosis of tumour of the colon is often made from the history alone and on suspicion. The patient is anaemic, has weight loss and intermittent constipation and diarrhoea, with the loss of blood or melaena per rectum. Barium enema usually confirms the diagnosis, but even in the absence of a positive barium enema, if the patient's history is characteristic, laparotomy should be carried out. Certain areas of the colon, notably the pelvirectal junction show up badly on barium enema and lesions here are commonly not shown. For these lesions at the lower end of the bowel the use of a sigmoidoscope is indicated and lesions up to 25 cms from the anus can be diagnosed by this means. Sigmoidoscopy also allows a biopsy of any dubious mucosa.

Tumours of Rectum

It is convenient at this point to consider tumours of the rectum. They are of similar type to those in the colon. Tumours in the rectum can be of the large fungating type or of the flat ulcerating type, but both produce characteristic symptoms in that the patient has diarrhoea and mucus per rectum with the passage of fresh blood. The diagnostic symptom is tenesmus. This is a feeling of incomplete emptying of the bowel. Following defaecation the patient immediately feels that he has not emptied his bowel and there is still something there to come away. This is due to the rectum interpreting the presence of the tumour as if it were faeces. Tumours of the rectum are easily diagnosed on rectal examination and confirmed by sigmoidoscopy. The treatment is to excise the rectum. If the tumour is high in the rectum, in its upper third, then the rectum can be excised via the abdomen and continuity of the bowel re-established by anastomosing the pelvic colon to the rectal stump. This is called anterior resection of the rectum. For a growth lower than the upper third of the rectum, however, the whole rectum must be excised and this is usually done by a combined approach from the perineum and the abdomen, the so-called synchronous combined abdomino-perineal resection of the rectum. This leaves the bowel terminating in the pelvic colon which must then be brought out in the left iliac fossa as a permanent terminal colostomy.

Preparation for Surgery

In the surgery of the large bowel the most essential factor for success is thorough preparation of the bowel beforehand. The bowel should be as empty and as clean as possible. The use of modern bowel sterilising antibiotics had led to the belief that if the bowel is sterilised surgery of the colon will be safe. This is quite false and in many cases has led to a worsening of the result because of the reliance on the antibiotic. There is no antibiotic which will completely sterilise the bowel and complete sterilisation of the bowel is not advisable as this will often allow an overgrowth of the fungi or yeasts which can lead to a fatal colitis. The most essential factor is mechanical cleansing of the bowel by the combined use of aperients and bowel wash-outs from below. The routine varies from hospital to hospital but a good routine is that two days before surgery an aperient is given, followed the following morning by an enema. The bowel is then washed out on the evening of the day before surgery and on the morning of surgery, and during this period the patient is given a low-residue diet to try and avoid faecal residues. In addition, bowel sterilising drugs may be given. These may be unabsorbable, (sulphonamides) and require 4—5 days before surgery in a very large dosage (16 Gm per day), or one of the anti-biotics. Their use has allowed quick bowel sterilisation. They are effective in 24—48 hours, the dosage being 4 Gm per day. The broad spectrum antibiotics, however, carry an increased risk of colonisation of the bowel by fungi and yeasts.

This mechanical cleansing of the bowel cannot be too strongly emphasised and indeed if at operation the surgeon finds much faecal material in the bowel he is well advised to perform a temporary colostomy rather than rely on his anastomosis standing up to the strain of the passage of hard faecal residues.

The patient may also require a naso-gastric tube to be passed into his stomach as this will help to cut down on the amount of post-operative sickness and also saves the patient's distress. The patient's skin requires to be prepared extremely carefully. The abdomen and chest should be thoroughly shaved and washed, the umbilicus must be clean and if the operation is one which will involve not only an abdominal incision but a perineal incision the patient will require the genital area, the anal region, buttocks and thighs to be thoroughly prepared and cleaned. The bladder must always be empty prior to surgery and occasionally if the operation to be performed is a very major one, a catheter may be passed into the bladder using an aseptic technique to prevent a post-operative retention of urine.

It is useful for the nurse to know what operation has been performed and to have a rough idea of what can be anticipated. The common operations on the colon are shown on the following diagrams.

Care after Operation

As many of the operations on the colon are extensive operations, the nurse must observe very carefully for signs of shock and to do this half-hourly recordings of the blood pressure and pulse will be necessary. Dressings must be inspected regularly for signs of bleeding. The patient will have an intravenous infusion of blood or fluid and therefore careful fluid balance chart must be maintained. Naso-gastric aspiration, either intermittent or continuous, will be carried out.

A short while after operation the patient will be commenced on small measured amounts of oral fluids which will be gradually increased

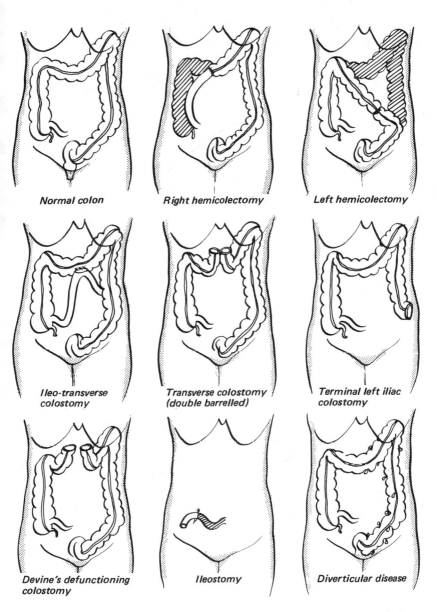

Normal colon

Right hemicolectomy

Left hemicolectomy

Ileo-transverse colostomy

Transverse colostomy (double barrelled)

Terminal left iliac colostomy

Devine's defunctioning colostomy

Ileostomy

Diverticular disease

183

in the same way as they are after operations on the stomach and duodenum until the patient is having a light low residue diet. If the bowel has not moved by about five days after the operation the surgeon may order a mild aperient or the insertion of suppositories. It is essential, however, that nurse does not stimulate the bowel except under very definite instructions from the surgeon.

After all resections of colon, whether the patient has had a colostomy or not, the motions can be expected to be frequent and soft for some time afterwards, since the removal of large areas of colon stop the re-absorption of water from the bowel and so the faeces are more liquid and defaecation more frequent. This, however, usually settles over the course of a month or two and the patient can be reassured that the motions should return in time to normality. There are, however, certain foods which tend to produce diarrhoea and to continue the frequency of bowel movements. These are best avoided, both in the post-operative phase and subsequently until the patient has confidence and can try them for himself. These are soups generally, but particularly those made with green vegetables. Also the pulses such as peas and beans and indeed any green vegetables. After the first few months, however, the patient can try these on his own and if he suffers no ill effects then there is no reason why he should not return to a full and normal diet.

The patient's sutures in his main wound will be left in for 10 to 12 days. If the patient has a perineal wound this will either be a cavity with packing inserted in it or a sutured wound with a tube drain in position. The packing would gradually be removed after 3 to 4 days and thereafter the cavity irrigated daily and allowed to heal slowly. Alternatively if the perineal wound is one with a tube drain the wound may be irrigated through this.

The specific care of the patient who has had an ileostomy or colostomy performed is considered in the following section.

The main complication of large bowel surgery, other than the complications common to all operations, is of leakage from the anastomosis. If this occurs soon after operation a very severe form of peritonitis occurs, although in the post-operative patient the signs and symptoms may be suppressed. More commonly, however, the leak occurs after several days and becomes walled-off to form a pericolic abscess. This commonly goes on to rupture, often in the wound or externally to form a faecal fistula where the bowel communicates with the surface of the body. Generally speaking, as long as there is no distal obstruction in the bowel this will heal spontaneously, but if the patient is severely ill, then a transverse colostomy is indicated to divert the faecal stream until the leaking anastomosis has had a chance to heal and fibrose.

After large bowel surgery patients will require convalescence and careful follow-up particularly when there is a malignancy.

Colostomy and Ileostomy

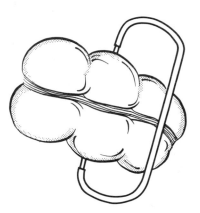

Loop colostomy showing colostomy rod in position

A Colostomy is frequently carried out as a temporary procedure to decompress an obstructed colon. In these cases it is commonly the transverse colostomy which is brought to the surface and is usually in the form of a loop supported on the skin surface by a glass rod or piece of plastic tubing.

In the obstructed colon which requires immediate drainage a cannula is inserted to allow gas and faeces to escape without contaminating the wound. This is removed in a few days time and the anterior two thirds of the circumference of the bowel above the rod opened with diathermy. In the palliation of unresectable tumours a similar colostomy may be fashioned and left unopened for several days to allow the wound to seal round the bowel. When these colostomies are opened there will be two openings, this is a double barrelled colostomy. The proximal opening will pass the faeces, the distal leads to the defunctioned bowel. The

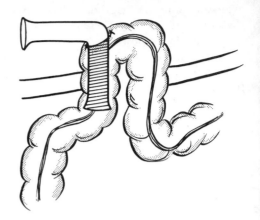

Loop colostomy — with glass tube in position for decompression

supporting rod is removed in 7 − 10 days.

Sometimes the surgeon considers it important to separate the ends of the bowel, e.g. in vesico-colic fistula so that no spill over of faeces can occur. In these cases the colon is divided at the time of operation and each end brought to the surface separately on each side of the mid line. The open bowel is usually sutured to the skin at the time of operation.

When the distal part of the bowel has been excised, e.g. in excision of the rectum, then a single open end of bowel is left. This is brought out and sutured to the skin as a terminal colostomy, usually in the left iliac fossa. In these cases there is of course only a single opening on the skin.

There are various appliances used to collect the faeces discharged from a colostomy. These belong to two basic types −

    1. Adhesive − where the bag is stuck to the surrounding skin or where a flange is stuck to the skin and disposable bags attached to the flange.

    2. Where a ring is held in place by a belt and disposable bags are attached to the ring. The type used will depend on the surgeon's preference and that most suitable for the individual patient.

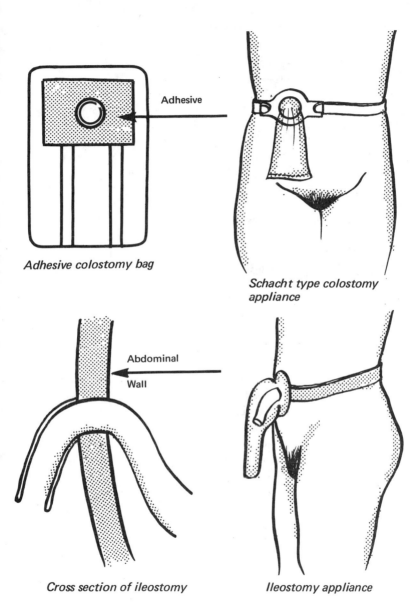

Adhesive

Adhesive colostomy bag

Schacht type colostomy appliance

Abdominal

Wall

Cross section of ileostomy

Ileostomy appliance

187

Since the discharge from a colostomy is formed and fairly non-irritant, the bowel can lie fairly flush with the skin. However, with an ileostomy the discharge is highly irritant and 5 centimetres or so of the bowel must be left protruding to form a spout and carry the discharge away from the skin and into the collecting bag. An ileostomy is required when the whole colon and rectum are removed for ulcerative colitis. Since it is the terminal ileum which is left the ileostomy will be placed in the lower right abdomen. It is usually made by bringing 7 – 10 centimetres of ileum through a hole in the abdominal wall and folding it back on itself to stitch the cut edges of the bowel to the cut skin edge. Thus the outer and inner layers of an ileostomy are covered with mucous membrane.

Appliances for ileostomies can be of similar types to those for colostomies, but the bags require to be more robust due to the increased volume and weight of the contents. It is better to examine the type in use in a particular unit than to attempt to describe them.

Care of Patient with Colostomy or Ileostomy

Before operation the patient would be given all the care already mentioned prior to large bowel surgery. The surgeon will discuss with and explain to the patient what is involved in his operation. He must be given the opportunity to express any worries or fears which he may have concerning it and nursing and medical staff may then be able to reassure him. It may be helpful either before or after operation if the patient could meet someone who has either a colostomy or ileostomy and is coping well and leading a normal life. The nurse must be aware that the patient may have tremendous difficulty in accepting what to him is a very dramatic change in his way of life and give reassurance and practical help as the need arises.

Colostomy

Post operative observation to make sure that the colostomy still looks healthy is essential. The skin requires much care to make sure that it is kept clean and barrier creams or ointments such as aluminium paste may be used until the colostomy has settled to fairly normal function Once normal colostomy function has been established cleanliness often suffices. The discharge from the colostomy may not commence until two days after operation but nurse should observe any escape of gas from the colostomy and she should also note and report when the colostomy first moves. Initially the discharge may be very fluid but as time passes it generally settles to a more formed consistency. It is initially cared for by the nurse who must not show any distaste at all when caring for it and must teach the patient to cope with all aspects of its care prior to dismissal. Once the colostomy has settled down it will act perhaps once or twice in a day. The diet initially will be of low residue but as the patient's general condition improves he can find out by trial and error what foods suit him and which ones he cannot take. It is generally advisable to have only a limited amount of roughage in his diet. The patient must be able to cope prior to dismissal and have all instructions regarding diet and colostomy care written down to give him something to refer to when he is on his own. He must, as with an ileostomy, know where to obtain supplies of dressings or equipment. This patient must return regularly to hospital for check-ups.

If the patient is using an appliance either for ileostomy or colostomy which involves the use of disposable bags, it is important that a check is made that the patient's home has facilities for their disposal. In view of the number of smokeless zones which have been created, many patients no longer have a fire in which they can burn things and only in the newest of the multi storey flats are there incinerators provided. If the bag with its contents does not float this can be flushed down the toilet. If, however, this is not possible the contents must be emptied into the toilet and the soiled bag wrapped very carefully in newspaper and disposed of in the outside dustbin. This latter method is not efficient or desirable and alternative methods should be sought for the patient. If this care is not stressed to the patient, particularly if they are in the older age group, they may collect a number of soiled bags before disposal. This obviously is completely undesirable and should be discouraged.

Ileostomy

On return from theatre the ileostomy must be carefully observed to make sure that it still looks a pink healthy colour. If it becomes discoloured it may mean that the blood supply has been obstructed and nurse must report this immediately. The discharge from the ileostomy may be very small initially but after about 24 hours and for the next 2 to 3 weeks the patient will have a very active discharge from the ileostomy. This is very upsetting for the patient and therefore she will require much encouragement and support from the nursing staff. After about three weeks the discharge should thicken a little and settle down to a smaller quantity. The discharge since it comes from the ileum will contain a lot of water and also some of the digestive juices. It is very important that the skin surrounding it is carefully cared for as these digestive enzymes and the presence of a lot of fluid could cause excoriation of the skin. The best way to prevent this is to keep the skin surrounding the ileostomy scrupulously clean. A well fitting appliance is another essential. The appliance will be chosen to suit the patient's needs and the nurse must make sure that it is also kept scrupulously clean at all times. It may be fitted on immediately after operation. The patient with an ileostomy will be given a diet which has a reduction in the amount of roughage and fatty fluids in it. Initially the nurse will be responsible for cleaning and caring for the patient's ileostomy and it is very important that she shows no distaste when attending to it. This can have an adverse effect on the patient and make him even more unwilling to accept his ileostomy. The patient should be encouraged as soon as he is fit to undertake the care of the ileostomy with supervision, and it is essential that the patient is adept at the care of it before he is discharged home. The Ileostomy Association is an association which exists to help people with ileostomies exchange ideas and to overcome problems. It is helpful if the patient has a visit from one of the members of the Association before discharge from hospital.

It is important that the patient has an adequate supply of bags and dressings prior to dismissal. The patient's General Practitioner must also be informed well in advance of dismissal so that he is acquainted with the patient's need of appliances and dressings materials and will be conversant with his difficulties. The patient must know at what chemists shops he may obtain the necessary items for his own particular care and this should be written down before the patient is sent home. This patient must return to hospital for regular checks. The patient should also be told on dismissal that if the ileostomy fails to work he must get immediate advice, particularly if he is feeling nauseated or has any pain.

28
Simple Conditions of the Anus and Rectum

Non-malignant conditions of the anus and rectum can be divided into painful and non-painful groups.

Painful Conditions

Anal fissure

An extremely common painful condition of the anus is a fissure-in-ano. This is a little split at the edge of the anus where the mucous membrane meets the skin. It is in fact just a tear of the mucous membrane, usually due to the passage of hard constipated motions. It is extremely painful and is often associated with bleeding. In acute anal fissure the treatment is to supply a local anaesthetic ointment to abolish the pain and sphincter spasm which accompanies it, although the basic treatment is to get rid of the constipation which initiated the condition and so mild aperients are given and the aim is to keep the motions soft, but not to produce diarrhoea. If the fissure has been present for some time, or if the local anaesthetic ointment fails to cure it within a period of 1 — 2 weeks, then further treatment is necessary. An injection of long-acting local anaesthetic can be made into the fissure to abolish the pain, but a rather better method of treatment is to stretch the anal sphincter under general anaesthetic until the anus will allow four fingers to enter. In a few cases, however, the fissure persists, to become thick-walled, fibrous, and chronic. When this occurs the only satisfactory treatment is excision of the fissure and this is usually coupled with division of the external sphincter muscles, known as a sphincterotomy.

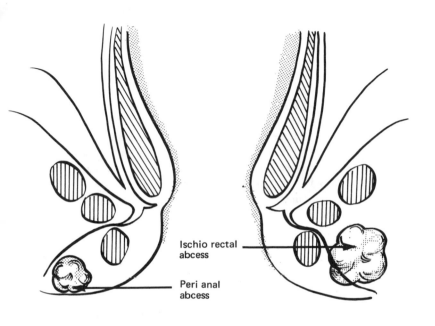

Abcesses of the perinium

Another painful condition of the anus and peri-anal region is peri-anal abscess. This area of the body is potentially always infected with the passage of faeces and the fact that the buttocks tend to seal off the space, and it is usually moist with sweat. Peri-anal abscesses may occur in the normal patient, but are extremely common in patients with diarrhoea, whether due to ulcerative colitis, diverticulitis, Crohn's disease, tuberculosis or the infective diarrhoea. The abscess may present to one or other side of the anus, rather like a boil, or it may occur inside the anal canal as a sub-mucus abscess. Occasionally the abscess may form deeply in the space between the rectum and the wall of the pelvis. This is known as an ischio-rectal abscess. These abscesses are extremely painful and debilitating and the treatment is the treatment of abscess anywhere — incision and drainage. If they are not treated promptly they may give rise to another very uncomfortable, painful condition — the condition of fistula-in-ano. If the abscess points and bursts on its own it may burst externally on to the skin, or it may burst internally into the rectum or anal canal. Not uncommonly it ruptures in both directions, forming a connection between the lumen of the bowel and the perianal skin. This is constantly exposed to the infective bowel contents and continuously discharges a little pus, is painful and uncomfortable and intermittently flares up into further abscess formation. The treatment of this condition is to excise the fistula and to leave it wide open to heal by granulation.

Pruritus Ani

This is the name given to a very debilitating condition where the patient has a severe itch in the perianal region. The basic cause of most cases of pruritus ani is an excessive mucus discharge from the rectum, which keeps the perianal skin moist and sodden. This may occur from any condition which irritates the anus or rectum, and commonly occurs in piles, fissure, fistula or indeed in constipation. Often secondary infection with fungi, such as monilia, occur, and this potentiates the pruritus, but in the majority of cases no satisfactory cause can ever be found for the itch.

Treatment in this condition is aimed at clearing up any local condition of the anus or rectum and by local medicaments for the skin. In the most severe cases it may be necessary to destroy the nerve supply to the perianal skin. This can be done by making an incision round the perianal skin and under-cutting it to raise a flap up to the anal margin and then suturing the skin back down again. If this fails then in the very worst cases it may be necessary to excise the perianal skin and apply a split skin graft.

Non-Painful Conditions of the Anus

Haemorrhoids

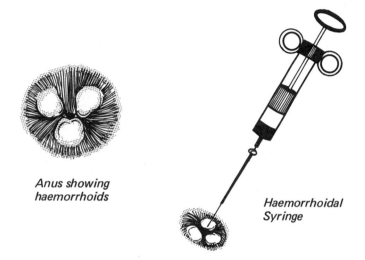

*Anus showing
haemorrhoids*

*Haemorrhoidal
Syringe*

These are one of the commonest simple conditions and yet one of
the ones productive of most misery that affects mankind, indeed it has
been said that the Battle of Waterloo may well have been won because
Napoleon was suffering severely from piles at the time and was unable
to control the battle adequately. So the course of history can be
altered by a simple anal condition. Piles in fact are varicose veins of the
venous plexus lying in the rectum. When viewed from below with the
patient in the lithotomy position these correspond to the clock positions
of 3, 7 and 11 o'clock. At first the mucosa covering the varicose veins
bulges into the rectum and then with the course of time enlarge and
they protrude through the anus, first of all during defaecation and then
eventually most of the time.

We divide haemorrhoids into three degrees.

1. First degree haemorrhoids are those which bleed on defaecation
   but do not prolapse outwith the rectum.

2. Second degree haemorrhoids are those which prolapse during defaecation, but reduce spontaneously at the end of the motion.
3. Third degree haemorrhoids prolapse and do not reduce and have to be replaced within the rectum manually.

In the uncomplicated state haemorrhoids do not cause pain. They bleed frequently and they cause a dragging discomfort in the anal region. They only produce pain if they prolapse and become obstructed outwith the body. This condition is known as strangulated piles.

The treatment of haemorrhoids is of two types. First of all, first degree piles are treated by local injection of a sclerosing agent, usually 5% phenol in almond oil and this can be guaranteed to stop the bleeding. Third degree haemorrhoids require treatment by operation, the operation being haemorrhoidectomy, where the piles are excised plus a wedge of perianal skin. Second degree piles, if they are mild, can be treated often by injection, but if they are severe they require haemorrhoidectomy, and it is often worth while to try injections in the first instance to try and avoid the operation; it is most unpleasant for the patient and most patients are terrified of it. When haemorrhoids become strangulated then surgery is postponed until the local condition has settled. The treatment is to put the patient in bed, raise the foot of the bed and try to reduce the haemorrhoids manually. If they can not be replaced, soothing solutions are applied to the part to shrink them so that they may be reduced manually, crushed ice can also be used for this purpose and causes some degree of local anaesthesia. Sometimes a stretch of the anal sphincter allows them to be reduced. Treatment should also include the avoidance of constipation, straining at the stool; and local medicaments while waiting for operation or during injection treatment may also provide great benefit. This can be in the form of an ointment inserted intra-rectally, or more commonly by the use of suppositories containing usually a local anaesthetic and some anti-inflammatory agent such as one of the steroids.

Anal Polyps

A common cause of confusion with haemorrhoids is the anal polyp. This is usually a simple adenoma of the rectum which, develops a stalk. This may protrude from the rectum during defaecation and may reduce itself thereafter. It commonly gives a feeling of tenesmus. The condition is easily diagnosed either by the use of the proctoscope or by the examining finger. The treatment is simple; ligitation of the pedicle and excision of the polyp. Occasionally these small adenomata, or adenomatous polyps of the rectum, can be a pre-malignant condition and they should be carefully examined histologically to make sure there is no malignant change in the base of the polyp.

Another type of papilloma that occurs in the rectum is the villous papilloma. This, unlike the simple polyp, is a mass of polypoid mucosa often covering a large area of the rectum. Its characteristic feature is that it produces a massive amount of mucus. The patient often complains of diarrhoea, but in fact is passing large amounts of mucus. This condition is often complicated by severe weakness, dehydration and collapse, due to the loss of large amounts of fluid and potassium ions which are excreted in the mucus. Although this is basically a simple condition it can become malignant if left untreated and should always be excised.

Familial Polyposis Coli

There is an uncommon condition where the whole colon as well as the rectum is involved with the formation of multiple polyps. This is a familial condition known as familial polyposis coli. It runs in families and its importance is this is undoubtedly pre-malignant and many of these polyps will become cancer if left intact. Treatment of this condition is a prophylactic colectomy once the condition is diagnosed. Most surgeons leave the lower end of the rectum intact so that the patient is spared the misery of a colostomy, but these patients must be followed up for the rest of their life with regular sigmoidiscopic examinations and any polyps recurring in the rectum should be diathermied immediately as they always carry the risk of malignancy developing.

There are also inflammatory conditions of the rectum, under the general term 'proctitis'. These do not themselves cause pain, but they all produce mucus discharge which tends to cause pruritus ani. Most of them are also associated with the passage of blood in the motions. One variety known as granular proctitis is in reality ulcerative colitis confined to the rectum and is treated by local steroids. Other types of proctitis are often non-specific where there is a diffuse inflammation of the rectum for no obvious reason, and the treatment again is by steroids.

Proctitis can also follow on irradiation of the cervix for carcinoma of the cervix in females. This is a particularly intractable form of proctitis, but the treatment again is by means of steroids locally.

Proctitis can also be associated with venereal disease. This only occurs in the female and is associated with gonorrhoea or lymphogranuloma venereum. The treatment is that of the causative disease. Occasionally, any of these varieties of proctitis may go on to form a stricture of the rectum. This presents as increasing constipation with the passage of ever-narrowing stools. Stricture of the rectum may be dilated with rectal dilators, or an incision may be made through the fibrous tissue to allow the rectum to dilate — the operation of internal proctotomy. Occasionally the stricture is so severe that excision of the rectum with colostomy requires to be carried out, or perhaps just the formation of a colostomy.

29
Jaundice

Jaundice is due to retention of bile in the blood stream. It gives rise to a yellowish colouration of the skin and conjunctivae, easily recognised clinically. Jaundice is basically of three types — haemolytic, toxic and infective jaundice, and obstructive jaundice.

In haemolytic jaundice there is excessive bile in the blood but the liver continues to excrete a normal amount so the faeces are a normal colour and there is no bile in the urine.

In obstructive jaundice the bile cannot reach the bowel and so the faeces are pale and classically described as clay-coloured, and bile is present in the urine giving it the colour of dark tea.

In toxic and infective jaundice elements of both are present giving a mixed picture.

Haemolytic jaundice is due to excessive breakdown of red blood cells.

Toxic and infective jaundice occur as a result of many bacteria and chemical poisons, and are most commonly due to a virus, causing infectious hepatitis. This can be transmitted in plasma and for this reason plasma as a substitute for blood in the treatment of shock is rapidly being superseded by synthetic substances. Haemolytic and infective jaundice are of more interest to the physician. The surgeon is primarily interested in obstructive jaundice.

In this condition bile is passed through the liver but is unable to enter the intestine due to some mechanical obstruction in the liver or the intestine. The common causes are

1. A stone in the common bile duct
2. Stricture of the common bile duct
3. Chronic pancreatitis, malignant tumour, most commonly of the head of the pancreas
4. Tumour of the liver

Pressure from without due to malignant deposits in the lymph nodes at the entrance to the liver can also obstruct the duct and cause jaundice.

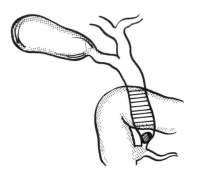

Stone blocking common bile duct

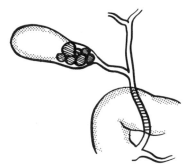

Stones in gall bladder

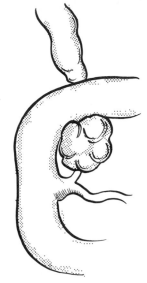

Carcinoma of head of pancreas

While the diagnosis of obstructive jaundice is fairly straightforward from the patient's coloration and from examination of the urine and faeces, the surgeon often wishes more detailed knowledge of the degree of jaundice and of the amount of liver damage. To this end he sends a sample of blood to the biochemistry department for a battery of investigations, known as the liver function tests.

The patient who is jaundiced has a variable degree of liver damage and in addition cannot absorb fats. The most important aspect of this defect is that the fat soluble vitamin K necessary for blood clotting is not absorbed and so there is a haemorrhagic tendency.

Since the treatment of obstructive jaundice invariably involves surgery, this clotting defect must be corrected before operation and therefore jaundiced patients before being submitted to operation must be given intramuscular or intravenous injections of vitamin K. They should also be given a low fat diet since fat cannot be digested in the absence of bile and they should be given a high carbohydrate diet since carbohydrate affords some protection to the liver against further damage.

The treatment of obstructive jaundice is to remove the obstruction and restore continuity of the bile passages. In the case of stone this is easily achieved by opening the common bile duct and removing the stones. If a stricture of the common bile duct is present then it may be impossible to widen the bile duct and repair it, and a by-pass operation may be necessary. In tumours of the pancreas or bile duct, removal of the tumour is commonly impossible and only palliative surgery can be carried out to relieve the jaundice by means of a by-pass. If the gall-bladder is present and if the cystic duct is patent, then the jaundice can be relieved by anastomosing the gallbladder to some suitable part of the bowel, either stomach, duodenum or jejunum.

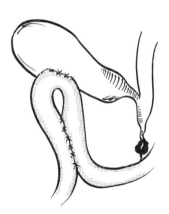

Cholecyst-jejunostomy
with enteroanastomosis

Apart from the conditions mentioned above, mild jaundice can occur in the presence of acute cholecystitis. The inflamed gallbladder leads to inflammatory changes and oedema and may lead to transient obstruction of the common bile duct to give a mild jaundice. As the cholecystitis subsides the jaundice will disappear. If, however, jaundice persists then exploration is necessary to establish continuity of the bile passages.

30
The Gallbladder

Gallbladder disease may be either acute or chronic. It is commonest in women who tend to be obese and who have borne children, but it can occur in young teenage girls. It is relatively uncommon in men.

In acute cholecystitis the patient has pain over the gallbladder region, i.e. just below the right ribs. There is a rise in temperature which is often quite high, up to 39·5°C, and the pulse is increased in rate. Vomiting is nearly always present. Most commonly acute cholecystitis spontaneously resolves with the giving of a broad spectrum antibiotic, rest in bed and light nourishing diet. If, however, the gallbladder contains stones then an abscess of the gallbladder may occur. This is known as empyema. In the worst cases of empyema, gangrene of the gallbladder may develop and the gallbladder may rupture into the peritoneum giving a very severe, and often fatal, variety of peritonitis. If empyema is suspected from the severity of the condition, from the high swinging temperature, or from a palapable, extremely tender gall-bladder, then operation should not be delayed. In these cases it is not uncommon for the operation performed to be merely a drainage of the abscess with insertion of a tube (cholecystostomy), since this will allow the patient to recover and the gallbladder can be removed at a later stage. Cholecystectomy in the presence of empyema or pus is often an extremely difficult and dangerous operation.

After acute cholecystitis the chronic disease may develop, although there may be several attacks of acute cholecystitis before the chronic form develops. More commonly, however, chronic cholecystitis occurs in the patient with gallstones. Here the symptoms are much less acute and the condition is one of flatulent dyspepsia. The patient has an aversion to fatty foods and suffers with marked flatulence and belching with a feeling of upper abdominal distension and a discomfort across the upper abdomen, particularly on the right side. Superimposed on this background of dyspepsia, there may well be attacks with fever, nausea and vomiting. The treatment of chronis cholecystitis is to remove the gallbladder (cholecystectomy).

In the investigation of gallbladder disease X-ray plays an important part. The x-ray which shows the gallbladder alone is called a cholecystogram, and consists of giving the patient a dye on the evening before x-ray. The dye is absorbed in the bowel and excreted via the liver to opacify the gallbladder. If the patient is then given a fatty meal, the gallbladder should contract and a further x-ray will show how well it functions in response to fat in the bowel. The cholecystogram may show the presence of gallstones, or may show a non-functioning gallbladder. This is the commonest finding in chronic cholecystitis. Non-functioning gallbladder is usually treated by cholecystectomy.

A cholecystogram can not be carried out in the presence of jaundice. Nor can an intravenous cholangiogram, which is an investigation to demonstrate the gallbladder and bile ducts, where, instead of taking tablets of the dye orally, the dye is injected intravenously at the time of the x-ray. This is used normally to show the bile passages, or it may be used where a cholecystogram has failed to give information about the gallbladder.

Gallstones

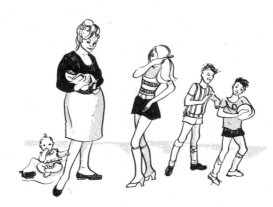

Fair Fat Forty Female and Fertile

Gallstones occur most commonly in women and are classically said to occur in women who are 'fair, fat, forty, fertile and flatulent'.

The presence of gallstones may produce no symptoms at all, since they are not uncommonly found in advanced old age in people who have suffered no serious inconvenience. They commonly, however, give rise to cholecystitis, either chronic or acute, and in acute cholecystitis, as mentioned above, may well precipitate an abscess in the gallbladder.

In the stones get into one of the ducts then severe pain is caused — known as biliary colic. This causes severe cramping pain in the right hypochondrium, commonly radiating to the back and to the right shoulder, and is often associated with the collapse of the patient. The pain does not last long and passes off only to come back again within a few hours. If the stone enters the common bile duct then it may obstruct there and give rise to obstructive jaundice. Occasionally, if the stone obstructs the duct at the entrance to the duodenum, bile may flow into the pancreatic duct, giving rise to pancreatitis.

The biggest risk, however, of gallstones is that they may give rise to cancer of the gallbladder. Cancer has never been described in a gallbladder which does not contain stones and it is generally assumed that the presence of stones in the gallbladder gives rise to chronic irritation which may predispose to cancer, and for this reason, apart from any other symptoms, a patient who is found to have gallstones should be advised to have a cholecystectomy.

Gallbladder surgery can be amongst the most difficult operations. Partly because the anatomy of the region is subject to great variation, but also because of the typical build of the patient the operation must be carried out at a considerable depth. Before operation the urine is tested for bile and nurse keeps a specimen for doctor. The stools must be observed for the colour and any constipation should be noted. If bile is flowing freely the stools will be of the normal colour. If, however, there is some obstruction to the flow of the bile the stool will be very light in colour. Vitamin K is one of the fat soluble vitamins and it is necessary for the production of the factors in the blood which allow it to clot. Bile is needed for its absorption so that the patient who is having an operation on the gallbladder, particularly if this has been preceded by jaundice, may be given injections of vitamin K before going to theatre to prevent haemorrhage after return from theatre. The patient may also have a naso gastric tube passed into the stomach to prevent post-operative vomiting and discomfort. After operation in the patient may have an intravenous infusion in position which will continue for approximately 24 hours. Within a few hours of operation the patient will be allowed some oral fluid and gradually by the third to fourth post-operative day the patient will be on a light diet. The naso gastric tube generally stays in position for about 24 hours. Vitamin K injections, if given before operation, are often continued after operation. The liver-bed normally oozes blood after this operation and it is not uncommon for the raw surface of the liver to drain bile for some little time. It is therefore a routine practice for a drainage tube to be left down to the gallbladder bed, brought out usually through a stab wound below the right ribs. This drain is left in position for 2 — 5 days, or until drainage is minimal. If stones are present in the common bile duct, or if the common bile duct is explored for any reason (choledochostomy), then T-tube drainage is normally instituted. Some

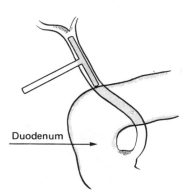

Duodenum

*T-tube drain in position in
common bile duct*

surgeons do close the common bile duct without drainage, but this is uncommon. A T-tube is left in the common bile duct with the arms of the T up and down the duct on either side of the incision and the T tube is brought out in the right flank. The bile is allowed to drain from this tube into a bag at the bedside. The T tube is only removed when the surgeon is certain that bile is able to freely re-enter the duodenum and when the tract along which the T-tube leaves the abdomen is sealed off from the peritoneal cavity. The T tube should never be removed during the first 5 days. To decide when the bile is flowing freely to the duodenum, an x-ray can be carried out (− called a T-tube cholangiogram −) where dye is injected along the T-tube and an x-ray will show it flowing into the duodenum if the passage is clear. A simple practical way of demonstrating free entry of bile into the duodenum is, starting about the third day after operation the tube is clamped for an hour the first day, two hours the second day, and the length of time it is clamped doubled each day until it is clamped for the entire day. If bile is entering the duodenum the tube is clamped without any upset to the patient. If the patient feels pain or discomfort, the tube is unclamped, doctor is informed and it is assumed that bile is not entering the duodenum. Most commonly a combination of the two methods is carried out.

Removal of a T-tube is uncomfortable and the patient must be placed in a resting position with a second nurse available to reassure her. A steady pull removes the tube but nurse must remember to cut the anchoring stitch before attempting to remove the tube. A small dressing is applied and nurse should expect a little leak of bile from the tract of the tube for a few days after it has been removed, but this should dry up spontaneously without further treatment.

Operations on the gallbladder and biliary tree are normally followed by nausea for a few days post-operatively. This can be very distressing for the patient, but can usually be easily controlled by injections.

The patient is generally allowed up to sit on the second post operative day and activity is increased until the patient is moving freely around the ward. The patient is normally allowed home after two to three weeks and should return for review. The patient is generally advised to have a holiday or a period of convalescence.

Gallbladder disease is commonly associated with hiatus hernia, duodenal ulcer and diverticulitis, and search for these diseases is always made during operations on the gallbladder.

31
The Pancreas

Diseases of the pancreas are not very common in this country. Infections of the pancreas may occur either in an acute form or in a chronic form and carcinoma may occur in the pancreas. Acute pancreatitis occurs as a surgical emergency where the patient is admitted shocked with severe upper abdominal pain and incessant vomiting and retching and closely mimics a perforation. The diagnosis is established by finding the amylase level in the blood to be raised. The treatment for this condition is not operative and is by means of intravenous infusion, suction, sedation and the giving of vagal blocking drugs to stop further secretion of pancreatic enzymes which are being liberated free into the peritoneal cavity.

Chronic pancreatitis, on the other hand, produces chronic illness characterised by pain, usually in the back, malnutrition often, indeed emaciation, and occasionally jaundice. It is extremely difficult to diagnose except by exclusion, for the pancreas does not show on x-ray, nor indeed are there any diagnostic tests. Treatment is varied and may involve widening the pancreatic duct where it enters the duodenum or excision of a portion of the pancreas.

Carcinoma of the pancreas is also an insidious disease causing back pain and emaciation. It commonly occurs in the head of the gland, where it results in obstructive jaundice. Curative operation involves a very major operation and is rarely possible. Usually a palliative by-pass operation to relieve the jaundice is all that can be done.

32
Hernias

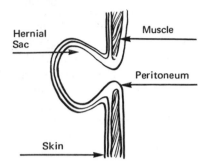

Cross section of typical abdominal hernia

Hernial Sac

Muscle

Peritoneum

Skin

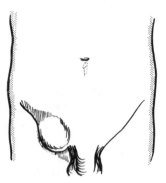

Right Inguinal Hernia

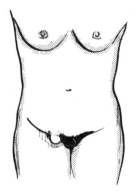

Right femoral hernia

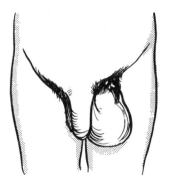

Left scrotal hernia

A hernia is the protrusion of the contents of a body cavity through a defect in its wall. When we speak of hernias, we tend to always think of hernias in the abdomen, but of course hernias occur elsewhere, e.g. the muscles can bulge out through a gap in the overlying sheath of the muscle, or indeed the upper part of the brain can protrude through a gap in the dividing membrane to enter the posterior part of the skull and this is a cerebral herniation.

However, the hernias which commonly require surgical treatment are those in the abdomen. Two factors are necessary for the production of these hernias

1. A weakness in the abdominal wall
2. Some increased pressure inside the abdomen forcing the contents out of it.

The weakness in the abdominal wall may be a congenital one, such as the inguinal and femoral canals. These are tracks extending through the muscles of the abdominal wall, the one from the peritoneal cavity to the scrotum (inguinal canal) which is created by the descent of the testes during foetal life. The femoral canal represents the track from the abdomen into the thigh through which the lymphatics from the leg reach the body. Other congenital orifices are at the umbilicus where the umbilical cord traversed the abdominal wall, and the oesophageal hiatus through which the oesophagus enters the abdomen. All of these form potential tracks for a hernia to push its way through. The weakness of the abdominal wall can also be acquired and the most common cause of this is following surgical operation. The scar is weak and may allow protrusion of the abdominal contents. This type of hernia is known as an incisional hernia or a ventral hernia, although it can equally well occur in the patient's side following an operation to remove a kidney when it is known as a lumbar hernia.

As well as the weakness in the wall, there must be increased pressure inside the abdomen. This may be due to some chronic condition, such as constipation or enlargement of the prostate where the patient has a strain to pass water or pass a stool. This constant straining increases the abdominal pressure greatly, or a chronic cough in the patient with chronic bronchitis raises the abdominal pressure. Other causes may be a large intra-abdominal tumour, or indeed the recurrent increase in abdominal pressure which occurs during pregnancy.

The hernia usually presents itself to the patient as an uncomfortable bulge at one of the sites mentioned. The pain is often described as being dragging in nature and is often such that the patient is unable to perform his daily work. The hernia is usually most prominent during straining or when the patient is ambulant and will often go away and disappear entirely when the patient lies down or is at rest in bed. Sometimes, however, when the hernia contains bowel the bowel becomes stuck in the hernia and cannot return to the abdominal cavity. When this happens we say the hernia is incarcerated and this leads to one of the complications and that is obstruction of the contained bowel. The major risk of herniation, however, is the risk of strangulation. This occurs when the blood supply to the bowel in the hernia is interrupted. When this happens the loop of bowel in the hernia becomes gangrenous, the patient becomes extremely shocked, shows all the signs of obstruction and vascular collapse, and will die if nothing is done to relieve the obstruction. A strangulated hernia is one of the most urgent cases demanding emergency surgery. For if operation is not carried out quickly the bowel may be entirely dead and have to be resected, or if delay is undue the patient himself may succumb.

This complication, however, is much less commonly seen now-a-days as most people have their hernias repaired as an elective procedure long before they get to the stage of strangulation.

The treatment of hernias is to replace the bowel in the abdomen to excise the sac of peritoneum which surrounded it, and to repair and strengthen the defect in the muscular wall of the abdomen.

Patients who have had repair of a hernia are nursed in the same way as any other patient. There is no need for them to be confined to bed for unduly long periods of time. They should be allowed up and about in the few days immediately following surgery. It is naïve to expect a stay of an extra 4—5 days in bed to contribute to the successful repair of the hernia. The patients are instructed not to lift heavy weights for several months after the hernia is repaired.

When hernias occur in the groin in men, they are commonly inguinal hernias, or in women rather more commonly they are femoral hernias.

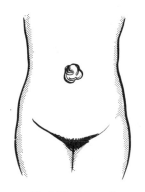

Umbilical hernia

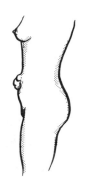

Umbilical
hernia
(lateral view)

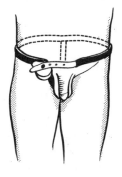

Truss for
inguinal hernia

A cause for difficulty in diagnosis in scrotal hernias is often the condition known as hydrocoele. This is a large fluid-filled swelling which occurs in the scrotum. When the testis descends into the scrotum it carries with it a sac of peritoneum. This normally shuts itself off from the abdominal cavity at birth, but a small pouch of peritoneum is left round the testis. This is continually secreting a little fluid which serves to cushion the testis. In the condition of hydrocoele the absorption of this fluid is interfered with and as it continues to be produced the little sac round the testis enlarges progressively, fills with fluid and may reach a relatively enormous size. This is most uncomfortable and causes a heavy dragging pain in the scrotum.

This condition, however, is quite simple and is dealt with by operation when the sac is excised.

APPENDIX

Operations on the Stomach

Partial Gastrectomy

Partial gastrectomy usually entails removal of the distal two-thirds of the stomach. The name given to the operation refers to the type of reconstruction. The prefix anterior or posterior means where the anastomosis is carried out in relation to the colon.

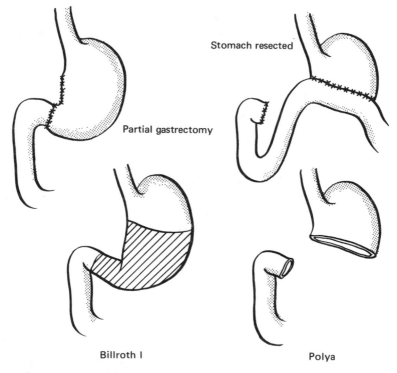

Stomach resected

Partial gastrectomy

Billroth I

Polya

Vagotomy

There are two vagus nerves, one anterior and one posterior. They supply the stomach in the main but the anterior gives a branch to the liver and gallbladder while the posterior gives a branch to the coeliac plexus to be distributed to the upper bowel. These branches are spared in the operation of selective vagotomy whereas in total vagotomy the whole nerve trunks are divided.

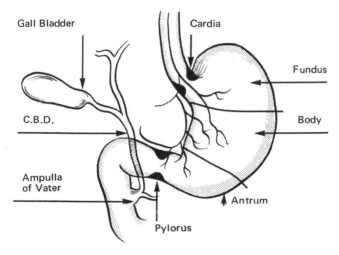

Areas of the stomach

Gastroenterostomy

This is the anastomosis of the proximal jejunum to the stomach. The peristaltic wave in the jejunum can run in the same direction as that in the stomach (isoperistaltic) or in the opposite direction (antiperistaltic). Again the prefix anterior or posterior refers to its relation to the colon.

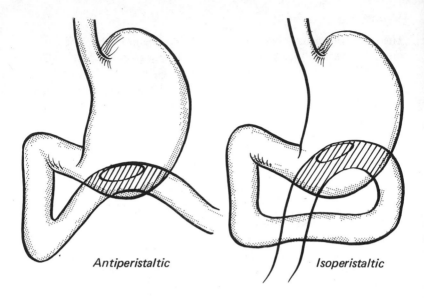

Antiperistaltic   *Isoperistaltic*

Pyloroplasty

A longitudinal incision in the wall of the bowel divides the pyloric
sphincter. The incision is then sutured transversely to further widen
the lumen of the bowel.

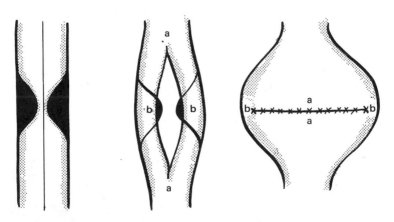

Total Gastrectomy

After total gastrectomy the bowel can be reconstituted using jejunum or colon.

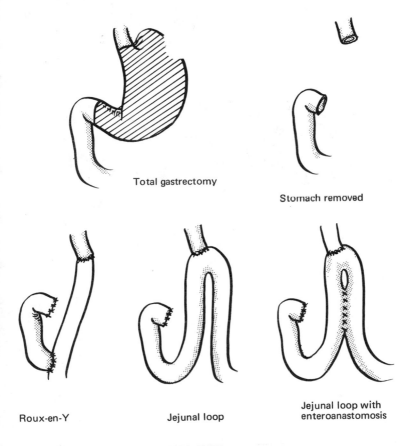

Total gastrectomy

Stomach removed

Roux-en-Y

Jejunal loop

Jejunal loop with
enteroanastomosis

Jejunal Reconstruction

217

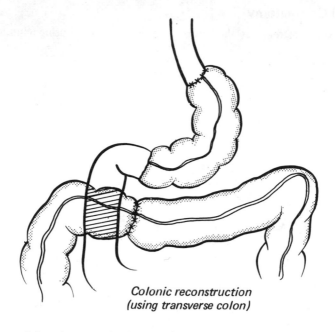

Colonic reconstruction
(using transverse colon)

Right or left colon can also be used in a similar fashion.

Preparation for X-ray Examination

Preparation for x-ray examination varies from one hospital to another. The following is suggested special preparation in addition to the routine for some of the commoner x-ray examination:—

Barium Meal, Barium Swallow and Barium Series

1. Nothing to eat or drink from midnight before examination.
2. If pyloric stenosis is queried — gastric lavage and drainage on morning of examination, and possibly a longer fasting period if desirable.
3. Aperient — night after examination.

Barium Enema

1. Aperient — 2 nights before examination — (Except when inflammation of bowel).
2. Low residue diet — day before.
3. Colonic Lavage.
4. *Tea and toast for breakfast and lunch on day of examination.*

Straight Gallbladder, Abdomen, Kidneys, Ureters and Bladder

1. Aperient — 2 nights before examination.
2. Low residue diet — day before.
3. *Tea and toast for breakfast on morning of examination.*

Cholecystogram (Tetra)
Straight x-ray of the gallbladder — day prior.

1. Aperient — 2 nights before examination.
2. Fat free meal at 6.30 p.m. on day before x-ray examination.
3. Telepaque tablet: taken half an hour after meal, i.e. 7 p.m.
4. No further food but fat free fluids may be taken as desired.
5. Cholecystogram 14 hours after the administration of the Telepaque.
6. *Tea without milk on the morning of examination.*

Intravenous Biligrafin (cholangiogram)

1. Aperient – 2 nights before examination.
2. Low residue diet – day before.
3. *Fasting on morning of examination.*

INDEX

222